# RESEARCHING WITH CARE

## Applying Feminist Care Ethics to Research Practice

Tula Brannelly and Marian Barnes

With a foreword by
Joan C. Tronto

P

First published in Great Britain in 2022 by

Policy Press, an imprint of
Bristol University Press
University of Bristol
1–9 Old Park Hill
Bristol
BS2 8BB
UK
t: +44 (0)117 374 6645
e: bup-info@bristol.ac.uk

Details of international sales and distribution partners are available at
policy.bristoluniversitypress.co.uk

© Bristol University Press 2022

British Library Cataloguing in Publication Data
A catalogue record for this book is available from the British Library

ISBN 978-1-4473-5976-0 hardcover
ISBN 978-1-4473-5977-7 paperback
ISBN 978-1-4473-5978-4 ePub
ISBN 978-1-4473-5979-1 ePdf

Cover design: Nicky Boroweic
Image credit: iStock / akiyoko

# Contents

# Notes on the authors

**Marian Barnes** holds the title of Emeritus Professor at the University of Brighton, UK. She previously held a chair in social research at the University of Birmingham. She has researched user involvement and user movements, citizenship and participatory democracy. Her later work focused on the ethics of care, ageing and wellbeing. Her many publications include: *Power, Participation and Political Renewal* (Policy Press, with Janet Newman and Helen Sullivan); *Caring and Social Justice* (Palgrave); *Care in Everyday Life* (Policy Press) and *Ethics of Care: Critical Advances in International Perspective* (Policy Press, with Tula Brannelly, Lizzie Ward and Nicki Ward).

**Tula Brannelly** is Senior Lecturer in Mental Health Nursing, Auckland University of Technology, New Zealand. Tula is a registered nurse, who has worked in practice, education and research with a long-standing interest in policy and practice influences on people who use services. Her research is often co-produced, and with marginalised groups, such as people with dementia, and she is interested in how people are subject to detention and compulsion without consent. Tula's research has used the ethics of care in analysis of professional practice and to guide research practice. Her publications include *Life at Home with a Dementia* (Routledge, with Ruth Bartlett), *Ethics from the Ground Up: Emerging Debates, Changing Practices and New Voices in Healthcare* (Bloomsbury, with Julie Wintrup, H. Biggs, A. Fenwick, R. Ingham and D. Woods) and *Ethics of Care: Critical Advances in International Perspective* (Policy Press, with Marian Barnes, Lizzie Ward and Nicki Ward).

# Acknowledgements

We would like to thank the people who have been part of our research, those with whom we have researched, and who have generously given their knowledge, time and care.

# Foreword

*Joan C. Tronto*

In this book, Marian Barnes and Tula Brannelly provide some guidance to researchers who wish to use care ethics as a guide to their research. As will become quickly apparent, this is not another book about research methods. Indeed, it is almost a book against such methods. As the American political theorist Sheldon Wolin warned, more than 50 years ago, even to think about 'methods' as the way to approach knowledge starts with some presumptions about the world:

> The kind of world hospitable to method invites a search for those regularities that reflect the main patterns of behavior which society is seeking to promote and maintain. Predictable behavior is what societies live by, hence their structures of coercion, of reward and penalties, of subsidies and discouragements are shaped toward producing and maintaining certain regularities in behavior and attitudes. Further, every society is a structure bent in a particular and persistent way so that it constitutes not only an arrangement of power but also of powerlessness, of poverty as well as wealth, injustice and justice, suppression and encouragement. (Wolin, 1969, p 1064)

In the ensuing decades, the quest for 'methods' has made the short path towards 'research' ever the more well-trodden. Every graduate student must now take at least one course in research methods, and scholars delight in producing tomes that make such lists. Throughout the leading institutions and processes of academia that today inform the global practices of research, a consensus seems to exist that good research can be measured by such markers of academic success as number of articles or books published, number of citations, and ranking journals and presses based on their popularity with other similarly situated researchers. The whole system seems to reinforce Wolin's concern that recreating and reflecting what is predictable and normal is the main purpose for scholarly work.

   The view of research presented here starts with a different premise and ends up elsewhere. It marks what Thomas Kuhn (1970) first called a paradigm change: a different approach to research. What marks this paradigm change for Brannelly and Barnes is that they begin from the premise that research should be done with care. And such research looks remarkably different. We can use Wolin's way of putting the question to see the basic elements of this alternative view. Wolin wrote, '[m]ethod is not a thing for all worlds. It presupposes a certain answer to a Kantian type of question, What must the world be like for the methodist's knowledge to be possible?' (Wolin, 1969, p 1064). And we might similarly ask here: what must the world be like for the caring ethicist's knowledge to be possible?

Since care aims at specific ends of making a world that is more hospitable to care, it is no surprise that the knowledge care scholars seek to create and find in the world is different. Perhaps no difference is greater than the difference in recognising the relationship between knowledge-seeker and the 'subjects' of their research. Because, indeed, even the language of research subjects already contains within it a hierarchy of researcher above the object of research. Rethinking research from the starting point of caring for what will be researched turns the research endeavour on its head.

Think for a moment about the nature of the 'research question'. The standard textbook on research methods tells researchers to start from a 'puzzle' and then to think about their 'data collection strategies'. But already the paths diverge. Is the research question coming from a 'gap' in the knowledge of the research community? If so, solving the puzzle is likely to result in a tidy publication. But if, as would happen in care ethics research, the question comes from the real life of some affected people, formulating the question might itself be more complex. Nevertheless, care ethics will provide a framework within which such questions take on meaning. The questions will be meaningful not because there is a gap in the literature, but because there is a real-world problem that requires solution. Choosing 'methods' for research will thus look quite different, drawing upon thinking through the issues the authors outline in this book.

Think for a moment about the ways in which the 'ethical' dimensions of the research emerge. In standard research, there are protocols issued by Institutional Review Boards (IRBs) that outline what ethical questions researchers should notice. But there may as well be deeper ethical issues involved that the IRB will simply miss.

Finally, think about the largest question, which emerges if we put the matter as Wolin does. What must the world be like for the caring ethicist's quest for knowledge to be possible?

It means that knowledge is not all the same – it is not all flat, dead, objective, there for the taking. People's knowledge, knowledge that is part of a particular community's heritage, for example, must be treated with respect, and not all of it might be available to everyone. Knowledge from different knowledge traditions may have other structures, and thus, from a standard research perspective it may not seem precise. And knowledge may originate not only from humans, even if the topic of discussion seems to be about humans. There may be stories that are complex and contradictory. Part of the researcher's task is always to sort through complexity. There is no easy 'method' here. After all, even in familiar forms of care, for example, when a parent cares for a child, the perceptions about what happens are likely to be different depending upon whose perspective is taken. As Brannelly and Barnes make clear, care ethics research requires an engagement with the messy realities of complex situations. Sometimes, as the authors make clear in the text, researchers will uncover details about organisations or movements that do not display them in the best light. Under these conditions, what should the researchers do?

Perhaps the most revolutionary claim here is about responsibility. If the usual paradigm presumes that researchers are merely observers of ongoing processes, then there really isn't much concern when they finish their research and move on to other topics. Researchers who do care-ethics research need to think about the effect that their research has on the others – human and beyond the human – who have been affected by their work. What is the proper care-ethical way to deal with the subjects left behind after a research study ends? Imagine a care project to design new architectural creations to see if people can care better in well-designed spaces. Who bears the responsibility for displaced residents? For the construction waste and noise generated in building the project? Care ethics requires that we understand the total context of research and its effects, and do not leave the consequences to someone else.

Since the type of knowledge that care ethics seeks to generate is knowledge that allows us 'to live in the world as well as possible', it is no surprise that such research is often oriented towards social change. And it is no surprise that it involves engaging research 'subjects' as co-investigators. Because their account of the *goals* of the research are also central to whether the research is going to succeed in living 'in the world as well as possible'. Such engagement cannot come from ticking boxes on a questionnaire at the beginning of a project.

It may seem that this form of knowledge and research are most appropriate in the human sciences. But it is also the case that such research can be useful in other contexts as well. In architecture, medical science, engineering, one can (and is sometimes professionally obliged, as for engineers) to perform one's work to meet 'standards of care'. The production of waste, for example, in creating new knowledge in natural scientific experiments has historically been treated as something that is outside and beyond 'the science' itself, but perhaps this perspective is wrong. Questions about responsibility for the effects of research clearly engage those in the natural sciences as well as those in the human sciences.

The final answer to Wolin's question, then, what must the world be like in order for knowledge that arises out of care-ethical research to matter, is complex and multifaceted, but clearly it is not the same thing as what is at stake in finding a literature gap to fill in with an article.

What the world must look like, then, to do research with care begins with the normative end, 'to live in the world as well as possible'. Some research cannot be done because it cannot be done, by these standards, in an ethical way. Some research, though, will yield great results in guiding theory and practice about care. Who defines what this will mean, how to resolve conflicts among different knowers and parties, how to engage in a manner that is respectful, all of these are serious matters of ethical research that this approach places at the centre of research work.

From the standpoint of this new paradigm of research, much of existing research, indeed many techniques of research, may appear to be lacking in their ability to provide useful literature. This would probably be a good outcome. When care ethics guides research, we can expect different kinds of research questions, different kinds of research outcomes. This new paradigm promises to upend academic practices that have lost their purpose and direction. This is, therefore, nothing but good.

Read and use this helpful book the way you would use a compass. You will not need to follow it at each step, but you will be able to return to it when you need to make sure that you are still headed in the right direction. The more caring we can make our research practices, the more we can generate the kinds of knowledge that will help us transform our world into one that is more completely committed to caring well.

# PART I

# 1

# Research and ethics of care

My research began with questions about voice: who is speaking, and to whom? In what body? Telling what stories about relationships? In what societal and cultural frameworks?

Carol Gilligan, 2011, p 5

This is a book about research – but it is not a book about methodology. We, Tula and Marian, are or have been researchers in academic settings who have researched with people directly affected by the topic of that research. Like Carol Gilligan, we have been concerned with questions about voice. Who gets to have a say about what is important to them? What happens when some voices are considered authoritative and others aren't? What happens to people when they are not heard or told that they are speaking in the wrong way? What about those for whom voice is not possible? And if we, as researchers, care about such things, what are the consequences of this for the way in which we approach our research and the responsibilities we carry for making a difference?

In this book we want to talk to people who do research as all or part of their work, and to those who may be invited to take part because of their membership of a particular community, because they share an experience, or because they use specific services. These latter groups of people are sometimes called 'experts by experience'. All those people may have an interest in research as a means to social change. So we want to consider what we research and why, and who makes those decisions. This book is about how we research, what we do to try to make a difference as a result of what we have studied, and who benefits from that. To whom are we accountable and who do we feel responsible for when we do research? This book also questions who are the 'we' who have appeared right at the start of our introduction. Who does social research and on what authority do they draw as they do so? How do those who do research relate to others who may be the subjects of research and whose lives may be influenced by what we do? Because we (Tula and Marian) think these are important questions to address we will tell you (the reader) something about ourselves and how we see ourselves in relation to the issues we explore in this book. We introduce ourselves briefly in this introduction and will say more at appropriate points as we develop examples and arguments throughout the book.

Like many of those who might identify themselves, at least in some contexts, as social scientists, we adopt a critical perspective on the questions we pose. But we are not interested in critique simply as a way of pointing to problems without any solutions, and we look to create new imaginaries and construct new possibilities from the work that we do. We recognise that even when research does offer new ways of thinking and new insights, this, too often, does not lead to real change. All those involved can experience frustration at the lack of change resulting from research. For research to be truly transformative requires us to move beyond critique to action, but we may be unsure how to achieve this. We have started with many questions and we do not propose to answer them all! One of the things we have learnt is that we need to be wary of certainty – in research as in other practices. We need to adopt a stance that enables humility and the capacity to learn from others, but we also need helpful ways of enabling us to reflect on questions we need to face up to as we carry out our work and, if we care about this, we need to ensure that what we do leaves things a bit better than when we started. We think that the ethics of care offers such a framework (Gilligan, 1993; Tronto, 1993, 2013).

So, this book is also about care. What do we care about and why? What does it mean to care about something and to spend part of our lives exploring those things we care about through research? How important is it to practice care in the research we do, in the way we relate to those we research with? How can we carefully try to use our findings to make things better? How do we achieve or at least travel towards progressive transformation that shows care to those involved in or affected by research? As well as drawing on the work of care ethicists we also draw on the work of Andrew Sayer (2011) to consider how social sciences cannot do other than to include care, to acknowledge that 'what matters to people' is central to understanding our lives as social beings. We draw on the work of Linda Tuhiwai Smith, an indigenous scholar in solidarity with decolonising research (Smith, 1999/ 2012) and how research praxis is concerned with humanness and interactions beyond the human (Kimmerer, 2020; Haraway, 2016). And we connect this to our own and others' work in care ethics to suggest what this means for the way we research together.

Tula and Marian met at the University of Birmingham, UK, in 1999. Tula was embarking on a PhD about citizenship and care for people with dementia, Marian was heading up research in the School of Applied Social Studies. We were both interested in and concerned about the way in which people with mental health problems experienced health and social care services, and excited by the way service users, survivors and disabled people were campaigners for social justice. Some of those activist groups had identified research as both a means of oppression and a site for change (Sweeney et al, 2009). We both worked with SureSearch – a group of mental health service survivors who researched with academics based in the university. When we discovered Selma Sevenhuijsen's (1998) work on the ethics of care we immediately recognised the power of this to draw out the tensions between calls for rights based in justice and calls for responses to need that were based in care and the necessity for caring relationships. This work helped us make sense of issues that both excited and troubled us about campaigning based in a claim for 'rights not care'. This had been a rallying call for some of those in the disability movement who had experienced being cared for as infantilising and disempowering and thus rejected 'care' as a basis on which 'helpful' support might be based (Shakespeare, 2000). While we sympathised with the social justice aims of the disabled people's movement, we were uncomfortable at the wholesale rejection of care. As it has developed, feminist ethics of care has taken up the challenge advanced by Gilligan (1993) to distinguish care ethics from justice ethics, but has also addressed both the relationship between, and necessity for, both care and justice (for example, Held, 2006) for the most marginalised of groups who do not have a voice.

We came to Carol Gilligan's foundational work later (this was originally published in 1982). Her articulation of the 'different voices' in which young people seek to explore and make sense of moral dilemmas as they try to find their places in the world reflected some of the troubling responses we had experienced in relation to different voices among service user activists, our own encounters with ageing, illness and mental health problems in those close to us, and other personal accounts of caring relationships (see Barnes, 2006). In different places and in different sociocultural and policy contexts we have continued our conversations about care ethics. This book reflects our commitment to the importance of talking together about things, as well as the value of weaving together ideas and experiences that have their origins in what might seem very different lives. We tell stories of our own projects, those undertaken with others, and we borrow the stories of others whose starting points are in other places in multiple webs of care when we think they help us deepen and expand the potential of researching together with care. Our focus is primarily on empirical research but we do not consider it helpful to think about research as being 'only' empirical or 'only' theoretical. So we include within our discussion work that might be defined as 'scholarship' as well as that which involves engaging with the messiness of empirical work.

We are writing at a time when optimism about progressive futures is hard because of a resurgence of populist politics, racist discourse and spiralling environmental catastrophe. In 2020 the COVID-19 pandemic caused us all to become more aware of both our vulnerabilities and interdependencies and has had a radical impact on how it is possible to conduct research. Ways of being and doing together that embody care rather than fear or hate require constant reinforcement and the necessity for such practices has never been more urgent. We do what we can, we sustain existing connections and look for new ones that can strengthen resistance, make modest shifts, enlarge and sustain the imagination necessary for renewal and transformation.

The feminist ethics of care is a critical approach that seeks to understand the necessity of care to wellbeing, to understanding marginalisation and identifying responsibility to remedy social injustices. From Gilligan's identification of the different voice of care ethics in comparison to justice ethics, it has gained traction as a critical perspective within many different scholarly and applied disciplines, as well as forming a basis for political analysis, environmental activism, health and social care practice and others. The boundaries that Joan Tronto (1993) sought to dismantle, between politics and morality, between public and private life, and the boundaries built on assumptions of a disinterested 'moral point of view', must stay down. Here we also explore other boundaries that thinking with care encourages us to look through and step beyond. We adopt an expansive view of care ethics, recognising that what it is, what it can be, is not determined by a view either from nowhere or a single somewhere. The necessity for care to be grounded in particular contexts requires us to consider care and care ethics as pluralistic, as demanding an attentive focus on both the who and the what we are interested in as we embark on doing research.

One particular way in which our thinking, and that of others, has developed, is the need to think about the limitations of the 'social'. If this restricts our thinking and our research to the solely human world, are we in danger of maintaining the damaging fiction that it is only humans that matter? Our current circumstances in the face of both environmental catastrophe and the impact of zoonotic disease mean we can no longer care about people to the exclusion of other matters of care (Puig de la Bellacasa, 2017). As social scientists we have had to fight to get our way of research accepted as respectable within cultures dominated by biomedical, physical and technoscience research. But can we any longer assume that wellbeing and social justice are achievable without including consideration of what is happening to the climate, to soil, to other-than-human animals, to biodiversity? We name human exceptionalism as another boundary that researching with care asks us to overcome. We reach out to researchers in other disciplines who understand and have demonstrated necessary interdependencies beyond the human, and we join with others who refuse to be bound by ways of thinking defined by disciplinary boundaries. Acknowledging interdependencies intends to situate humans within the complex and messy realities of life and recognise the interconnections and relationships that are present in social research and between social and other sciences, arts and humanities.

Caring requires thinking about knowledge just as much as research does. Knowledge is as contested a concept as care. Dalmiya (2016) argues that knowledge is not possible without relation and that knowing is fundamental to caring. Wilful ignorance is a position that lacks care. Being open to new evidence and ways of knowing and actions of actively seeking new knowledge shows care. Openness requires capacity for seeking new knowledge and the willingness to move reflexively with it. Knowledge and knowing is always partial as it is impossible to know all of another's experience (Visse and Abma, 2018). In the same text, Hamington (2018) reminds us that care is a form of inquiry, and to care deeply requires in-depth knowledge, that knowing is to care as care and knowledge are intertwined.

Our exploration of the practices of research lead us into thinking about how we know and how we think. Care ethics and participatory methodologies have developed side by side over the past years (Brannelly, 2018). The ethics of care asks us to think about our relationships with others, particularly those made vulnerable by different forms of oppression or marginalisation. So too do the challenges to researchers from participatory and co-productive research methods (Reason, 1994; Banks et al, 2018). Such methods aim to include the voices of people who have been silenced, muted or devalued. They offer challenges to assumptions about hierarchies of knowledge and methodologies for generating this. They link research to action and remind us of our responsibilities to those who may have been harmed by research in the past. It is significant that when disabled people, survivors of mental health services and others who have used health and welfare services developed their own research projects and methodological approaches they drew from feminist research that both values experiential knowledge and seeks to challenge marginalisation and oppression (Rose and Beresford, 2009). This connection between the ethics of care and participatory approaches to research is one that has also recently been made by Alena Sander in her work on Jordanian women's organisations (Sander, 2021). Our (authors) experiences of researching with and being challenged by disabled and survivor researchers has been enriched by drawing on feminist scholarship on care ethics, on new materialism and post-humanism as well as feminist methodologies. We have also learnt from the work of indigenous researchers who offer a distinctive perspective on what epistemic injustices mean and on human/other-than-human relationships. We try to reflect some of this in the sources we draw on throughout this book. This book shows how the ethics of care provides a systematic approach that supports researchers and communities to make sound judgements about research practices and claim further ground to see meaningful impacts from research. Objectives are real-time changes for marginalised communities, in solidarity with community aims.

Much of what we write about in this book comes from what we have learnt as we have tried to research *with* rather than *on* people. It is also a response to what we think is a corruption of both the principle and the practice of co-production in research. Researchers seeking funding in the UK are asked to say how those with experience of the topics to be researched have been involved in developing the proposal, and how they will be involved in carrying out the work. Too often this has led to box-ticking consultation with those invited into research as consultants, peer researchers or other 'active participants' having unrewarding experiences. But it also recognises that many of those who do research feel troubled and lack confidence about how to resolve what seem to be contradictory pressures to research in ways that are both respect-able and respect-ful. As we recount stories of projects from different perspectives later in this book we will consider the troubles many feel. Resolving troubles may be neither possible nor desirable. Our aim is to offer ways of thinking, doing and reflecting together in research that can sustain connection rather than exacerbate conflict and resentment, even when genuine differences remain. Our reflections and conversations with novice and seasoned researchers identify moral dilemmas and challenges that arise during research that are often minimised and seen as unconnected, yet every research study has them. Researchers are concerned that they are not showing due care to people involved in their studies. They can feel that they are inadvertently demonstrating a lack of care and respect by minimising opportunities to guide the research, or by interpreting what is said through their frame of thinking, rather than recognising this as an alternative view. Inadequate time and resources can be given to hearing the voices of contributors, and to creating space for change within the project. Accounts of such troubles and their consequences are usually only offered publicly when they are significant enough to derail a project. Researchers feel they are expected to be on top of all aspects of their work and to admit to disagreements or uncertainties among those involved can be seen as failure. We need to be prepared to offer accounts that reflect different experiences and challenges, and that identify the moral and emotional work that goes into researching with care.

Researching with care can be understood as a response to the failure of methodology to ensure inclusive participation is offered to the people affected by the issues that are researched. Gilligan's identification of a different voice in moral decision making resulted from her recognition that girls and women were excluded from psychological research which theorised human development (we discuss this in more detail in Chapter 3). We expand that insight to consider other exclusions from research and the range of different voices we need to hear to understand and transform the world. To do this we need to care about those who are excluded and seek ways of bringing in many different voices. We need to recognise research as one of the 'things we do' to live in the world as well as possible (Tronto, 1993) and so to craft research practices that embody care ethics. Visse and Abma (2018) grapple with similar concerns in their text on evaluation practices and theory, *Evaluation for a Caring Society*. They recognise people as evaluative beings who notice when care is absent, that care as an unfolding praxis requires exchanges and reflection, and that creative practices enable good storytelling and sharing. These sentiments are rarely present in the theoretical or practice discussions about evaluation of policy and practices in which marginalised voices are present.

In our own research we have worked primarily with people who, because of illness, disability, age or emotional distress, have needed to enter into relationships with health, social care and welfare services. In Tula's case, some of this work has been with those also experiencing the consequences of colonial domination of indigenous peoples. We recognise in our personal lives the way in which some experiences have a more than professional meaning for us. We are not only researchers, but women, growing older. We are daughters, sisters, friends who encounter the impact of ageing, illness and vulnerability in our personal lives and the lives of those close to us. Care ethics asks us to look at the different contexts in which care is given and received and refrains from offering a blueprint of how to act. Participatory research involves people with different relationships to care as well as to each other and leads to conversations about experiences that are both shared and unfamiliar. We will tell stories of research that seeks to care and to build solidarity in different conditions of being and becoming. As we tell these stories we reflect on the nature of story itself – are the stories told to researchers so very different from the stories offered in political testimonies or in literary accounts? And we wonder about individualism and the way social science pushes people to offer individual accounts that the researcher will aggregate in ways they determine rather than ways those being researched might desire.

Caring about exclusions and finding ways of doing research that demonstrate care in practice, applies the ethics of care in the field of research. We consider work that takes care ethics into worlds other than health, welfare and social care, including in environmental action and activist roles undertaken as part of research cultures. As we enlarge our conceptions of the 'we' who seek to live in the world as well as possible, and unsettle assumptions that it is only humans who matter so that we include animals, plants, soil and 'things' within the moral sphere of a web of care, we confront questions about the interaction between wellbeing and relatedness to the non-human world and what this means for participatory research. The unequal impact on humans of climate change and environmental breakdown is a matter of social justice as well as care. But environmental justice asks us to look in different directions. Politically, in terms of our very survival, we can no longer assume that transformations benefiting humans is enough. Not caring about the non-human world is no longer an option.

All research has, embodies and communicates assumptions, meanings and values about the natural, technological and social worlds. In this text, we draw on powerful accounts of critical care approaches that have identified and led to revisions of knowledge in the social and natural sciences. The necessity and science of contributions of indigenous knowledges are recognised. Intersectional approaches to inclusion are championed that enable researchers and communities to come together to express concerns and motivations that bridge experiential understandings with theoretical and empirical scientific work. Therefore, this text is intended for audiences beyond social scientists, and we aim to speak to anyone interested in taking an approach that can lead to change that can help us to live in the world as well as possible. Many researchers are motivated by a desire to improve the situations they research but lack guidance about how to create partnerships that enable short-term and longer-term change as part of research practice, or how to demonstrate and recognise the effect of participatory research methodologies. We hope to contribute to learning about how that can happen.

Fisher and Tronto's definition of caring is the starting point for this discussion:

> On the most general level, we suggest that caring be viewed as a species activity that includes everything that we do to maintain, continue, and repair our 'world' so that we can live in it as well as possible. That world includes our bodies, our selves, and our environment, all of which we seek to interweave in a complex, life-sustaining web. (Quoted in Tronto, 1993, p 103)

But we want to make a small but important revision to this trigger for much work on the ethics of care. That is the insertion of the word 'together' in the definition: 'to live in it *together* as well as possible'. This reflects Tronto's later addition of solidarity in the integrity of care. This focuses attention more directly on the necessity of interdependence and the essential relatedness of care. And that 'together' encompasses not only those humans whose voices and ways of speaking may be different from each other, but also entities that have no voice in the way that humans understand this. We also recognise the significance of temporality. We should not limit what we mean by 'living well together' to those who occupy the world within the same time frame. Relational interdependence encompasses the inheritance of ancestral relations that shape responsibilities in the present, as well as our responsibilities in the present to those unknown others who will come after us. Young's (2011) 'social connection' model of responsibility for justice enables us to both recognise past harms and to accept responsibility in the way we look forward to the future (see also Barnes, 2018). We consider that care-full research can help us make those temporal connections.

From the Fisher and Tronto definition of caring, we also give more scrutiny to the concept of 'repair'. Both of us have written about care and transformation, while others have suggested that the concept of repair is too conservative to serve the progressive claims that care ethicists have made. But while progressive movements counter the exclusions and silencing experienced by disabled people, indigenous people and others, and in doing so may argue that there is not a 'whole' state to which to return, we argue there is a need to recognise the damage that has been done by different forms of injustice and to repair this. In the way that we research with people we need to understand the consequences of exclusions and silencing, and to recognise the brokenness of personal and social relationships resulting from those processes. One of the things that is purposive about caring in research is that we seek to repair that damage. That means that how research is done needs to be informed about power relationships and the potential for the reproduction of oppression, including how communities who are marginalised have experienced research relationships in the past. There is a need to counter a 'progress' narrative, by providing a 'progressive' narrative that surfaces the tensions between progress and sustainability, including the more-than-human world not only as context for human caring relationships, but as implicated within a web of care necessary for sustaining and nurturing us all.

This text develops and extends the premise of care-based methodologies to inform research that builds on care ethics and care-based epistemologies. We argue that the ethics of care provides a systematic framework for researchers to reflect on research practices as they occur, critique how research projects respond to communities of involvement and inform a review of structures that support the achievement of the aim of reducing inequalities and promoting social justice. Just as we cannot view knowledge as effectively generated from a single perspectival position, care necessitates conversations and dynamic reflections involving those occupying different positions within caring relationships. Researching with care includes deliberation as an aspect of research, considering the relationships in which research is embedded, how marginalisation and inequality are framed and presented, and evaluation with people affected by issues under investigation to ascertain whether careful research has been achieved. We explore what this means in practice as we offer accounts of different projects and researchers' reflections on their own practices and the troubles they have experienced. We look at how researchers practice humility and tact in research relationships and how these are at odds with the academy's expectation of expertise and persuasion.

Part I of the book engages critically with care ethics as a framework for research practice by examining the roles of assumptions, emotions, meanings and values in the production of knowledge, what we mean by relational care in research, and the transformational opportunities possible through an ethics of care approach. The second part of the book is more descriptive. It draws together accounts of careful research practices, reflections on the challenges and troubles of those undertaking this kind of work, and guidance for ethical research relationships. It addresses contentious research issues in practice, how it can be possible to build solidarities and create change, including through a commitment to support activism in communities. The final chapter provides an overall reflection on an ethics of care research systematic approach to guide research from initial ideas, through doing research in practice, to the ways in which those involved seek an impact from the work they have done.

## Book structure and chapter outlines

### Part I

Chapter 2 focuses on knowledge, emotions and values in research of all kinds, including studies of policies and organisations as well as social relationships and everyday life practices. We challenge the possibility of value-free research, including research from positivist paradigms, and then we turn attention to the tendency of social sciences to decontextualise research to a degree that the meaning can be lost. To do this we draw on the work of Andrew Sayer (2011) and his critique of how social science research that edits out what people care about produces knowledge that is disconnected from everyday life, a limitation of academic endeavour. An examination of values and their influence on knowledge is necessary for a critical approach that considers power and has the aim of achieving social justice.

Our starting point is that people research what they care about. Most people involved in research do so because they feel some connection with the research area. There is reason to celebrate the connectivity that people have to research, but this has frequently been named as a 'problem'. Researchers are urged to create distance, maintain objectivity and avoid emotional engagement. In this chapter we introduce how this has implications for the way that participatory methods are practised and corroborates the frustrations that are frequently reported in research collaborations. Good research practice contends that the experience of end users of the research is utilised in the design of all kinds of research to inform an approach that affords better research questions, recruitment strategies and communications with service users and others affected by the research topic. In a health context this recognition has led to a surge in 'public and patient involvement' that has inevitably led to variable practices from researchers alongside the creation of a group defined as 'experts by experience'. This new set of actors in research understand the variability of research collaborations and commitment to impact and action.

We work with a broad definition of social science research as the study of society and how humans influence the world around us. This reflects the extensive uptake of ethics of care in diverse disciplines including environmentalism, human geography, business management, law and international relations. We also consider the interaction between social science and work within the humanities, in particular philosophy, literature and other arts, that helps us recognise and include different ways of storytelling and meaning making within our repertoire of participatory research practices. We discuss indigenous knowledges and scientific approaches that ask critical questions of the purpose and role of research in the future of the world. Attention is drawn to the varied and multilayered types of knowledge including experiential, theoretical and praxis, and their place in care ethics thinking. This, and our discussion of the importance of experiential knowledge, is one way of posing questions about how social scientists might collaborate with researchers in other traditions or in novel and interesting spheres of research, for example through interspecies approaches. The ontology of interdependence and interconnectedness is more than metaphor. We reflect on the relationship between values, meaning and assumptions and the influence this has on the production of knowledge in different scientific arenas. The ethics of care is a situated moral philosophy. It encourages us to break down the barriers built up through containing different disciplines within separate silos.

In Chapter 3 we deal with two central tenets to the argument of this book: that research is both relational and political. People do things to and with other people in research settings. We ask questions of others intended to find out about experiences that may be unfamiliar to us. How we frame those questions may have been influenced by others who have had similar experiences in order to ensure that questioning is carried out as sensitively as possible. Often, the people who are the focus of research are marginalised in some way, they may have been treated badly by services ostensibly intended to help them. Previous experiences of oppression and hurt may frame thinking about participation in research projects, for example with indigenous communities for whom research may be experienced as a re-enactment of colonisation. We revisit Carol Gilligan's (1982) ground-breaking work which involved girls and young women as well as boys in research about moral dilemmas and thus both questioned and expanded theories of moral development. This provides a springboard to consider the relational in research, and how research is political and personal. It also highlights the emotional work attached to research and research relationships. In a more recent turn, Donna Haraway (2016) has challenged conventional thinking about research and social action in the post-human world and the responsibilities of interspecies research. Her story of working with pigeons as researchers on a project about air pollution illustrates the possibility of careful cross-species collaboration. In this chapter we start to draw out the moral responsibility that researchers have for both the way they conduct research and for its impacts. How often do researchers consider responsibility? Research exposes power relations, difference, diversity and connections. These are surfaced and exposed through the doing of something together, and may be challenging and conflictual and deeply personal.

We also discuss the limitations of 'problem' based research, based on categorical definitions that constrain matters of concern and interest. Intersectionality requires us to be careful about assuming identifications based in one aspect of identity and calls on us to think about dynamic relationships within the research process. This intersectional approach acknowledges power in the lives of research participants and the political implications of becoming involved in research and political action. It also challenges the claim that only certain people may research certain experiences and instead calls for ethical approaches to research that is sensitive to the particulars of positionality. We intentionally blur the boundaries between the accepted categories employed to operationalise research (to funders and ethics committees for example) to acknowledge that we are not only researchers or research participants, but occupy and negotiate different aspects of identity as we work together. In a critical engagement with the literature on emancipatory and participatory research methods, aspirations and challenges to achieving emancipation in research relationships are reviewed with reference to the constraints and opportunities offered by stakeholders such as institutions and funders.

Chapter 4 is about researching with care. We start with a justification for approaching research as an activity that we can think of as 'care', then move to a more detailed discussion of what research practices that seek to embody Tronto's phases of care can look like. Applied to research, Tronto's phases of care include attentiveness to all involved, responsibility to research participants and others, competence to carry out research well, responsiveness from others to actions, and solidarity as an aim of research practices. These phases can guide as well as critique and review practices, and question the aims and outcomes of research in terms of what happened, what was accomplished and for whom. We offer examples from our own work and that of others that illustrate this.

The ethics of care definition offers 'repair' as an activity of care, and in this chapter we look at the ways that social research can fulfil the need for repair through research relationships that are attentive to people who face oppression in the current, past or future. Recognising that oppression carries harms and damage from the present into the future provides the context in which research relationships start. But it is also necessary to understand research relationships as a continuation of relational care or abuse predetermined by prior inherited relationships. We call on research to 'show love for future generations' (Edwards et al, 2020; www.indigenous.ncrm. ac.uk/resources/), a consideration used by indigenous communities when considering whether to allow access to communities.

## Part II

We start the second part of this book with introductions to six other people who have been involved in various ways in researching with care. In preparation for this part of the book we invited them to have conversations with us about their work, to talk about some of those issues that often do not appear in published outputs from research, and to offer their reflections on care ethics in research. We are grateful to these people for being prepared to share their experiences with us and to use these in this book. The following three chapters develop our considerations of what researching with care means in practice by drawing on these different experiences, alongside some of our own, to consider how we start out on research (Chapter 5), how we work together in the process of doing research (Chapter 6), and in Chapter 7, how we approach analysis and try to secure positive change as a result of our work. The final chapter draws together the arguments throughout the book and offers overall reflections on the value of ethics of care thinking in guiding and reflecting on research practice.

Chapter 5 is about how to reach a decision about what needs to be researched, who may be involved in that decision, and what influence this has on designing a research project. Asking people what they care about, what matters to them, can be a helpful starting point and a reminder that the world can look very different to those who are differently positioned in relation to the research topic. People care about topics for different reasons, but as researchers explore these issues, they can become more aware of what drives their own interests and where it is important for them to acknowledge that a lack of knowledge can result in unhelpful assumptions. We recount stories of researchers being surprised, becoming more aware, recognising that they needed to rethink their approaches as a result of their early encounters with people involved in the initial stages of planning research. This can involve both conceptual rethinking and a need to work in rather different ways in practice if the experience of taking part in research is to be a good one, and the outcomes are to be experienced as beneficial.

The attentiveness that is necessary in the initial stages of planning and designing research continues throughout a project. In Chapter 6 we examine the *doing of* research in partnerships from an ethic of care perspective. Here our focus is on the process of research, but we argue that we need to avoid a binary distinction between process and outcome, not only because learning comes from process, but also because the experience of taking part can leave as much of a legacy as what are more usually considered 'research findings' can achieve. So here we expand on our consideration of research as relational practice by recounting both the joys and troubles of novice and more experienced researchers as they have sought to generate knowledge and understandings with others in different contexts. Working with others in the doing of research can ask us to be open to rethinking the language we use and the way we frame our ideas throughout the process. This can be particularly important when we are working in cultural contexts different from those with which we are familiar. A capacity and willingness to attend to how others respond to the way we present ideas demonstrates that we care about those with whom we work and encourages them to stay involved. But researching with care also means accepting our responsibilities to care for those we are working with. This can involve practical supports: arranging transport for old people to get to research team meetings, for example, as well as the provision of careful supervision of people who may have been confronted with unexpected and upsetting experiences in the course of the work. Our conversations with researchers working on different topics in different contexts enables us to offer a range of examples of what care for others in research means in practice. Done well this can facilitate the generation of new kinds of knowledge and can generate solidarity that in itself is a legacy of the research.

The ethics of care offers a framework which we can use to analyse and interpret data and, through its normative purpose, to 'renew' our understandings of what things might look like if approached with care. In Chapter 7 we offer examples of applications of care ethics to analysis, including Trace, developed by Selma Sevenhuijsen (2003) to interrogate policy documents. In line with our overall approach in this book, we also discuss careful analysis where the process of making sense of data is carried out in a collaborative way. Drawing on our own work and our conversations with others, we offer examples of what this involves in practice, and consider some implications for what is prioritised and presented in research outputs. We recognise the impact research has on those who take part in this and how the process of taking part can change us. It is important to seek good endings for our research together and to recognise the different parts of our lives that are impacted by this. We cannot expect others to make changes as a result of the work we do unless we ourselves are also open to learning from this.

In the final chapter we offer a series of questions that we think are helpful in preparing people to undertake careful, thoughtful research. We do not propose a specific methodology for researching with care, but rather encourage all those involved in research to think about the relational context in which they work and what this means for how they work together. We offer personal reflections on what care ethics has meant to us in our work and in our lives more broadly, noting the impossibility and unhelpfulness of trying to draw boundaries between the personal and professional as well as the personal and political. We also reproduce a poem by indigenous scholar Linda Tuhiwai Smith that offers a powerful reminder of why we need to both understand the damage that research has done in the past and the need to be careful about the legacy we leave for the future.

# 2

# Caring, knowing and making a difference

People who do research care about what they research. The topics they research matter to them, and how they impact on people matters too. Researchers live in relation to others in friendship groups, families, local or national communities, and through identities based in ethnicity, gender, sexuality, religion or other characteristics. They may choose to become involved in research to address the hardships or inequalities they see through personal experience, such as of racism or colonial domination; as a result of professional awareness, such as that of unequal access to health services or the impact of contemporary lifestyles on the environment; or through a political sense of injustices deriving from poverty or discrimination. Researchers may be connected to their research field in multiple ways, and the focus of their research may change over time as they start to become aware of other concerns (Letherby, 2003) and as they deepen relationships with those whose lives they research. Recognition of the positioning of researchers and their personal and political stance in relation to issues is quite common in social science circles, but it applies to researchers in all fields of enquiry. It is impossible to consider an environmental researcher who does not care about the state of the planet, or medical researchers unconcerned about finding cures or treatments for illnesses affecting people.

Researchers are social beings implicated in the world they research. In the introduction to his book *Participation in Human Inquiry*, Peter Reason (1994) made a similar connection to that we have been advancing between Fisher and Tronto's inclusion of 'repair' in their definition of caring; the practice of research, and the importance of thinking together the human and more-than-human world:

> I have been much persuaded over recent months by the image of the purpose of human inquiry not so much the search for truth but to *heal*, and above all to heal the alienation, the split that characterizes modern experience. … To heal means to make whole; we can only understand our world as a whole if we are part of it; as soon as we attempt to stand outside, we divide and separate. In contrast, making whole necessarily implies participation: one characteristic of a participative world-view is that the individual person is restored to the circle of community

and the human community to the context of the wider natural world.
(p 10; emphasis in original)

This participative worldview and the research practices it gives rise to are
what we want to explore. How researchers care about research is evident in
the stories they tell about their work, the emotional connection that comes
through when researchers explain how the area became of interest to them,
and what transformations were achieved (or not) through research projects.
Feminist methodology has given particular attention to how people are
connected to research (for example, Letherby, 2003). Feminist researchers
have encouraged researchers to reflect on their choices about what to research
and to write themselves into the research in order to acknowledge the
significance of the positionality of the researcher in relation to the researched.
In some instances, for example in the practice of critical autobiography (see,
for example, Church, 2004), this can be one and the same.

So our consideration of the ethics of care and research starts from the
recognition that people engage in research because it matters to them. This
applies both to those who undertake research because it is their job, and
others who might become involved because a project directly affects them
in some way. Research of all kinds involves processes of meaning making,
hermeneutics and evaluation. It is hard to think about how we might study
social structures, the way organisations operate, how services are delivered,
or how people try to care for each other, without at the same time needing
to understand what these things mean to people and what importance they
have for people's lives. Our thinking here is influenced by Andrew Sayer's
(2011) book: *Why Things Matter to People: Social Science, Values and Ethical Life*.
Sayer's approach to social science is that it must start from the recognition
that people are evaluative sentient beings, whose evaluations provide a guide
about flourishing and suffering that informs all of our lives. Sayer points
to the problem of scientific understandings editing out normative practical
wisdom, and thereby losing sight of what and to what degree different things
matters to people. This renders scientific knowledge as lacking practical
purpose, and misunderstands personal relations to research of the people
involved in it. In this reading of social sciences, any commitment to impact
is lost. Research is an end in and of itself, an academic practice that is not
concerned with change. But this is at odds with the motivations of many
of those involved in carrying out research and many of those who agree to
take part in it. It is a distanced view that creates a situation where personal
knowledge, experiential understandings and the insights of those directly
affected by what is being studied are viewed as biases rather than strengths
that can inform research practices and outcomes.

Sayer's characterisation of social science is important for this text as it
raises fundamental questions about the purpose of research. It suggests how

creating knowledge is an act that can distort social life to an extent that it no longer connects to people's concerns, and therefore is unable to add practical guidance for social change. What matters to people is formed from the moral and ethical sensibilities that people apply to everyday situations. Sayer argues that, in its focus on description and explanation (theory), social science has become separated from more philosophical approaches to the normative questions that are important in our everyday lives. What matters to people can be thought of as challenges to wellbeing. Wellbeing is relational, contingent on the quality of relationships we have with others, including how we experience respect and support (Barnes et al, 2018). Wellbeing is also dependent on our evaluations of external influences on flourishing and suffering. This connection between morality and wellbeing is largely ignored in a social science that prioritises interpretation through theoretical lenses. The removal of evaluative and emotional forces that affect wellbeing precedes a misunderstanding of social life.

The normative gap that can be produced by some approaches to social theory decontextualises moral problems into components that no longer make sense. Sayer's (2011) critical realism challenges constructivist interpretations and leads to a discussion about what counts as knowledge. Focusing on theoretical interpretation can blur the lens through which problems are viewed so that the experiential component that was vital to the research in the first place recedes from view. Whatever the orientation of the researcher in terms of their approach to research, the academy itself demands disciplinary interpretations that inadvertently deny the realities of research participants and thus result in an adequate representation of everyday ethical sensibilities. Sayer (2011) calls for post-disciplinary perspectives that overcome what he calls the 'tiresome disciplinary imperialism that is institutionalised in the academic division of labour' (p 248). These perspectives are evident in feminist post-materialist methodologies that reject the privileging of human exceptionalism and of dominant western epistemologies (Haraway, 2016; Ahmed, 2017). We also advocate for approaches that democratise research (Edwards and Brannelly, 2017), which are not bounded by disciplinary constraints, encompass knowledges other than those deriving from western scientific methods, and which recognise the importance of care as both practice and value.

The feminist ethics of care values practical wisdom (Barnes et al, 2015). Care is purposive and care-full research will both ensure experiences of oppressions, marginalisation and injustice are placed at the centre, and that just outcomes are sought from its findings. We argue that the opportunity to do research is a position of privilege that brings with it responsibilities. But accounts of responsibility and what this means for research and researchers are rarely included when findings are presented. We acknowledge our own shortcomings in this respect. One question that care ethics prompts us to ask is whether positions of privilege to conduct research are used for social good: how researchers can avoid perpetuating the privileged irresponsibility that Tronto names as one means of denying the significance of care (Tronto, 2013) and Zembylas et al (2014) point out is a violation of all elements of care. In the research context, avoiding privileged responsibility means creating change that supports good research through attentiveness, and sees that commitment through to the legacies of research partnerships.

## Meanings, values, knowledge and emotions

Accepting that we cannot understand social life without taking ethics and values into account does not mean assuming that we are dealing with things that are solely personal or subjective (Sayer, 2011, p 27). How and what people value; and what experiences, events and relationships mean to people is mediated through, but not determined by, social values. When we use concepts in research, we need to be aware of the implicit messages they convey and the normative statements they make about what is important. This is not just a question of how we use concepts in framing research questions. What matters is communicated by the ways in which decisions are made about what is important to research, what aspects stand out for investigation, and who should be involved in the research.

The dominance of positivism in research led to binary distinctions being made between 'facts' and 'values'. We, as many others learning how to research, were taught of the need to distinguish the two when seeking to generate 'evidence' from research projects. Andrew Sayer again:

> The view of values as beyond reason is part of a whole series of flawed conceptual distinctions that obstruct our understanding of the evaluative character of everyday life: distinctions such as fact and value, is and ought, reason and emotion, science and ethics, positive and normative, objective and scientific, body and mind, animal and human. (2011, p 4)

Single disciplinary positions call for clarity of perception through a singular interpretive lens applied to a clearly defined concept. Ingenuity of procedure may be thought of as the best method available to gain access to the data required to build knowledge. But clarity of perception potentially brackets out and devalues the messiness of life that feminists have argued better represents life as it is actually experienced and lived. Different approaches to methodology can be seen as ways of reintroducing the messiness of thought, belief, action, emotion and value that make up the way we live together and in relation to the natural and technological world. Examples include narrative approaches (Reissman, 2008) that focus on what we can learn and understand from the stories that people tell about their lives, and participatory methods that draw out the complex concepts and associations that people use to make sense of the world and their place within it.

Starting from the stories that people tell of their lives shifts our perspective from the conceptual and theoretical purity demanded from a monodisciplinary approach. Interdisciplinary or post-disciplinary approaches foster multiple perspectives and encourage attention to be given to the connections and relationships between people, things and ideas. Some of the most creative approaches to research not only use concepts from different social science disciplines – recognition of the value of taking account of emotions within analysis of economic decision making, for example – but also bring together both ideas and people whose starting points are in very different worlds. Some collaborations also encourage us to expand the way in which we think about what constitute the boundaries of research itself. An example of that is the way the artist Olafur Eliasson has collaborated with chronobiologists (who study biological time and the rhythms of our bodies and behaviour), architects, chefs, economists and others to create art that is also experimental research that not only explores relationships between light, space, environment and migration, but also the interaction between viewers, institutions and what happens when we see art together (Godfrey, 2019).

## Diverse knowledge

Research is intended to improve our knowledge. But as we have already hinted at, we need to embrace an expansive understanding of what knowledge is, as well as how it is generated and enhanced. The question of knowledge has itself been interrogated from many different perspectives and disciplines. Philosophers, social scientists, psychologists, policy analysts and others have considered how we 'know' and what is considered legitimate or credible knowledge. Writing during the COVID-19 pandemic we have been exposed to glib assumptions from politicians that 'the science' is uncontentious and that policy decisions informed by this will self-evidently be 'right'. Scientists aware of the potential for negative reputational impact have sought to distance themselves from political decisions, and the unfolding of the pandemic has revealed how partial and contingent scientific knowledge often is. Disagreements about what constitutes 'evidence' on which to claim robust knowledge is at the core of disputes between methodologists, not least those adhering to quantitative or qualitative methods. But it has also been fundamental to the challenges offered to 'professional' researchers by others who have been subjects of/subjected to research, and whose lives have been impacted by the authority claims of particular types of scientific endeavour. So we need to look at some of the ways in which what knowledge is and who is recognised as a credible knower have been debated. Our focus is on what type of knowledge has achieved legitimacy, how that relates to who is recognised as a credible knower, and how that, in turn, relates to issues of care and justice.

We can identify four different ways in which the relationship between knowledge and justice has been considered. Each recognises power as a key to understanding the dynamics by which types of knowledge and types of people achieve dominance and we can see intersections between them. However, because their starting points differ, they highlight the different mechanisms to which we need to be attentive when approaching ways of doing research with care.

Shiv Visvanathan (2005) writes about 'cognitive justice' from a perspective that views western technoscience as part of the process of the domination of colonised peoples: '[O]ne has to realize that epistemology is not a remote, exotic term. It determines life chances. Science as development, plan, experiment, pedagogy determines the life chances of a variety of people. Here epistemology is politics' (p 84). He notes that, in India, critiques of science did not emerge from disciplinary conflicts within academia, but from grassroots struggles among human rights activists, feminists and ecologists. His concern is 'knowledge transfer', and the assumed beneficial effects of introducing knowledge generated from within western knowledge systems and applying this to 'development problems' within very different contexts. He identifies examples of development projects that failed because of the way they ignored or marginalised the culture and knowledge of tribes, slum-dwellers or peasants. The harmful effects were profound: 'What was destroyed was not only the forest but a common body of knowledge about trees, fodder, forest produce, seeds, medicines, building. This was not merely a resource pool but a way of life that sustained knowledge' (p 89). Thus for Visvanathan, participation or community involvement is not enough to ensure a just democracy. Cognitive justice requires cognitive representation in spaces of policy making, 'the constitutional right of different systems of knowledge to exist as part of dialogue and debate' (p 92).

Since Visvanathan wrote about colonial domination and injustice through the imposition of a particular form of knowledge, both indigenous and feminist post-materialist scholars have argued for and practised with ways of thinking, writing and researching that reject such injustices. In the case of indigenous scholars the knowledge built up over centuries that has been obscured, undermined and dismissed has become more visible to those of us educated according to western 'enlightenment' principles. In different ways and in different contexts the connection between how research is conducted and how both particular groups of humans as well as the more-than-human world have been subjected to injustices has become more evident and the damage that has been caused has become more evident. While it remains the case that indigenous knowledges remain marginalised and risk continuing displacement and colonisation (Rosiek et al, 2019), the work of people such as botanist and citizen of the Potawatomi Nation Robin Wall Kimmerer (2020) offers inspiration by showing the link between indigenous and 'scientific' knowledge about plants, and how weaving such knowledges together can offer a way to counteract the damage we are causing to our world. Like Visvanathan, Kimmerer's understanding of the connection between the destruction of a particular way of knowing and the dangerous loss of environments necessary to sustain human as well as plant life, alerts us to the vital connection between knowledge, justice and care – for the environment as well as for other humans.

While Visvanathan focuses on the role of colonial domination in marginalising knowledge systems, philosopher Miranda Fricker (2007) addresses the role of prejudice in rendering certain 'social types' as lacking credibility as 'knowers'. Her primary focus is on gender and race and the 'identity power deficits' experienced by women and Black people that render them less trustworthy and believable because of the operation of stereotyping. Those processes engender what Fricker calls primary and secondary harms that are both sources of injustice:

> The primary harm is a form of essential harm that is definitive of epistemic justice in the broad. In all such injustices the subject is wronged in her capacity as a knower. To be wronged in one's capacity as a knower is to be wronged in a capacity essential to human value. (Fricker, 2007, p 44)

What Fricker also calls 'dishonouring' leads to a number of actual and possible material disadvantages. These include not being believed in a court of law and hence being more likely to be convicted of a criminal offence, and being at a professional disadvantage because of being seen to lack the judgement and authority required for promotion to senior positions. Fricker also suggests that the longer-term consequences of repeatedly being disbelieved can result in undermining a person so that she effectively 'loses knowledge' (2007, p 49). She identifies two forms of epistemic injustice: testimonial injustice that 'excludes the subject from trustful conversation' (2007, p 53), and 'hermeneutical injustice' which she identifies as a form of structural injustice that obscures from view experiences for which there is no name and thus are not seen to exist. She offers the example of women's accounts of behaviours to which they could not give a name, that have subsequently become recognised as experiences of sexual harassment. Fricker identifies Carol Gilligan's (1982) work in identifying a 'different voice' in ways of expressing ethical judgements as reflecting another example of how certain groups have been marginalised from practices within which meanings are generated.

These processes of undermining credibility, depriving a person of confidence in themselves as a knowing subject and being marginalised from those spaces and practices within which meaning is generated, applies, albeit in rather different ways, to people regarded as lacking capacity because of mental illness, learning or other cognitive difficulties. This is the third context in which issues of power, knowledge and ethics need to be brought to attention. It intersects with the fourth perspective which is that of the claims to authority and expertise based on exclusively held professional knowledge. In the contexts with which we are most familiar that is most obviously the case in relation to medical knowledge.

People living with mental health challenges are familiar with the experience of not being listened to; not being believed; being considered incapable of knowing what is wrong; 'lacking insight'; of being too confused to offer a credible account (see examples in Sweeney et al, 2009). While presenting findings of a study carried out with service users of experiences of being compulsorily detained in psychiatric hospital (Barnes et al, 2000), Marian encountered a psychologist who seemed unable to grasp that what was being described was participatory research carried out by academics *with* service users. He could not get beyond asserting that it was impossible to give weight to people's accounts of what had happened to them when they were sectioned (compulsorily detained in hospital under the Mental Health Act) since those accounts would have been filtered through disordered thinking. Such responses are perhaps more fundamental than stereotyping. They associate lack of credibility as knowers to the nature of a condition, which is itself used to identify people. Someone may be described as 'having cancer', but another as 'being a schizophrenic'. The characteristic of 'mental disorder', by definition, results in a lack of credibility. For those with learning difficulties it is an issue of 'mental capacity' rather than disorder that undermines recognition as credible knowers. While there are, of course, differences of degree and there have been significant changes in the extent to which people have been recognised as both knowers and experts in their own lives, it is still important to be attentive to the harms that have been done by failures to include people in processes of knowledge generation, and to acknowledge the inequalities in authority afforded to those whose expertise derives from professional training and those for whom it comes from lived experience. We know, from Barnes et al (2000) and others, that good experiences of inclusion can be part of a process of healing for those involved.

The intersection of personal, political and professional takes on considerable importance in this context. While it is entirely possible to be both user of mental health services and a worker in the mental health system (Barnes,

2015), separation between professional expert and 'patient' are written into the codes of diagnostic manuals which are the source of authority to name certain symptoms as evidence of disease rather than behavioural difference. Those manuals provide the evidential authority for diagnoses that have substantial impacts on the lives of people who become psychiatric patients. But their influence extends beyond the consequences of clinical intervention. Kutchins and Kirk (1997) recount the way in which psychiatrists were called to offer opinions on the possibility that Anita Hill, who in 1991 in the United States accused Justice Clarence Thomas of sexual harassment, was suffering from delusions. One introduced the idea of 'erotomania', which, although not substantiated, served to discredit Hill's testimony. This case offers an example of the discrediting that Fricker writes about in relation to gender and hermeneutical injustice intersecting with apparently 'objective' diagnostic categories. Another example of ways in which knowledge, gender and psychiatric diagnoses intersect in undermining women's credibility emerges from Anne Figert's (1996) fascinating, and at times humorous, account of disputes over the inclusion of pre-menstrual tension as a diagnosis in DSM-III/IV.

In a rather different context, care ethicist Eva Kittay (2010) recounts the story of her challenge to fellow moral philosophers who did not see a lack of knowledge about the lives of people with severe cognitive disabilities as an impediment to their assumptions about comparative moral agency. Their argument that cognitively disabled people had less moral agency than certain animals was extremely hurtful to Kittay as the mother of a daughter who is disabled. She urged her colleagues, at the least, to epistemic modesty before drawing conclusions about the lives of people with whom they had no familiarity. The connection between power, knowledge and ethics is one that researchers who aim to take a care-full approach to their work need to have at the forefront of their thinking and action. We need to be attentive not only to the individuals whom we encounter in research, but also to the different dynamics that inscribe differential credibility to both knowers and knowledge systems on the basis of what can be disputed categorical distinctions, stereotypical assumptions and a legacy of domination and injustice.

## Emotions

Closely associated with unequal judgements about people as credible knowers based in identity and cultural difference is the mode in which people speak and express their ideas and experiences. It is not a matter of chance that both women and people of colour have been seen as less credible: their capacity to convince others – White men – is constrained not only by being charged, in the case of women, with the sin of 'intuition' (Fricker,

2007), but in both cases by allowing emotion to trump reason in substance and expression. Kittay (2010) reflected on how troubling it felt to her as a professional philosopher to include her own emotional response in her argument with colleagues.

The most frequently acknowledged way of thinking about emotions in the context of research recognises that experiences such as those of illness, of ageing, living in poverty, of being sexually abused or racially oppressed, generate distressing emotions. These can include fear, guilt, shame and hopelessness, as well as anger. Researching lives that include these emotionally charged experiences asks people to recount stories of harms experienced and damage caused. Formal research ethics procedures ask those proposing empirical research in these and related topics to say how they will minimise distress and respond to it if/when it emerges during the study. But we cannot exclude it. Emotions provide important information about what matters to people, and what particular experiences mean to them. Martha Nussbaum (2001) argues that it is mistaken to regard emotions as 'non rational' as they have complex cognitive structures that express the relationship between the person and the object about which they are expressing emotion.

In the case of participatory research where those who know what it is to live with such experiences participate as co-researchers, researchers are frequently advised to only invite those who are considered to have 'worked through' their personal emotions. This is assumed to be necessary to enable them to deal objectively with the issues that will arise. But how *all* those who take part in research are able conduct themselves in a way that recognises the importance of such emotions without causing further harms is vital to care-full research. Making differential judgements about capacity for objectiveness and the priority accorded to an objective stance (where objectivity is seen to require a non-emotional rationality) among all those involved in conducting research could exacerbate harms already experienced. People living with mental health problems have spoken of the way in which any expression of emotion on their part can be pathologised. They are not allowed to feel 'fed up' without this being described as being in a 'depressive state', or to be excited without attracting a label of mania. But what about 'righteous anger' at the discrimination they experience?

The relationship between politics and emotions has been considered in relation to both mainstream politics and social movement action (for example, Goodwin et al, 2001; Clarke et al, 2006). Political action can be motivated by emotions such as anger at injustice; compassion for the circumstances of others; guilt or remorse at wrongs done – or even despair that things can change (Hoggett, 2006; Thompson, 2006; Cunningham, 2012; Gould, 2012). It can enable negative emotions such as shame to be transformed into positive emotions such as pride (Whittier, 2001). Participation in collective action can involve considerable emotional labour and be sustained by the emotional benefits received by the participants. Honneth's (1996) theoretical work on recognition underpins some of this more applied work and offers us one way of thinking about the importance of researching together as a means of achieving recognition and building solidarity (we develop this in Chapter 4). Here we need to note that emotions can motivate researchers who have different relationships to the subject matter, and that doing research can generate different kinds of emotions among those carrying out the work as well as those who are being researched. Thus, attending to the ways in which interviewees might respond to questions posed during research interviews is only part of the matter of being careful with emotions in research.

Doing research may make emotional connections with researchers' own lives that can be unexpected and unsettling. Kathryn Church describes such an experience as she worked on a doctoral research project with psychiatric survivors. As well as discovering the helpfulness of feminist theory in illuminating the practical dilemmas she faced in this project, Church faced a personal crisis:

> [T]he relationships which I formed with psychiatric survivors over the course of events had a remarkable effect: they cracked me open as a person. In seeking to understand survivor pain and politics, I plunged headlong into my own. Right in the middle of my research I experienced a physical and emotional breakdown. (Church, 2004, p 2)

The possibility that researching with others can unsettle separations between researchers and those they are researching or researching with, reflects the importance attached to attending to research relationships. Research projects create spaces in which intersectional identities are constructed, negotiated and challenged. How this happens and what consequences there are for both the research and for those taking part in it requires us to be careful about how we work together.

## Whose knowledge counts in research

Research is thus a site for contention over what counts as knowledge, who counts as an authoritative knower, and how research practices might engender both positive and negative responses to the possibility of creating new types of knowledge. Gaining control over the conduct of research became one of the objectives and strategies of the disability movement (Barnes and Mercer, 1997) and of the mental health user/survivor movement (Sweeney et al, 2009). Some drew a distinction between emancipatory research that had a clear political objective and was controlled and carried out by disabled people or survivors, and participatory research that involved collaborations between academic researchers and people with lived experience. The question of who should be involved in carrying out research is connected to the question of what kinds of knowledge are recognised, valued and included. Citing Haraway's claim that 'reality is an active verb', Puig de la Bellascasa makes the connection between the impossibility of knowing and thinking without the multitude of relations that make that possible, and the relational ethics of care: '*relations of thinking and knowing require care and affect how we care*' (2017, p 69, italics in original). Who we research with matters, and so does how we do this. Social researchers have sought to change research practice and build knowledge with people affected by the issues they are studying, but this approach and the incorporation of experiential knowledge is not always readily accepted. And acceptance does not necessarily mean that the practices adopted enable those involved to feel cared for, or that the process leads to the changes they hope for.

In this section, we consider how far we have come from the distanced, removed researcher magnifying, scrutinising and delivering knowledge from a singular point of view, to the challenges of multiple perspective, post-disciplinary research that has evolved to examine complex and interdependent webs and systems. We advocate a position that, reflecting the ethics of care, puts experience at the centre and values multiple perspectives that enable complex, messy and situated knowledge building with the potential to achieve change. At its best, participatory or co-productive research pursues these aims and goes some way to repairing harms. But it is not always like that.

If we look at participatory research in the health and social care context we can unpack some of the challenges experienced and faced by those wanting to work in this way. In the UK there is now an expectation that the voice of experience is present in any project undertaken. There is a broad continuum of what involvement may look like, from user-led research, where the lead researcher has experience of an issue, to consultation with people with experience to inform a bid application or as advisers through the project. Major health and social research funding bodies support projects that have an element of experiential knowledge threaded though the design. This call for involvement has generated a proliferation in user and carer groups who can play such roles within universities. As the approach has matured, so too has the critique of involvement and consideration of what constitutes meaningful involvement in research, and the capacity of researchers to facilitate good involvement. Workshops and seminars have sprung up to inform researchers about best practice and what may be experienced as poor involvement (see, for example, Banks et al, 2019).

In order to achieve the transformative potential of working with experiential as well as academic or theoretical knowledge, people need to be involved at the right times. Both what things mean and how things matter need to be up for discussion and negotiation throughout the research. Ethical and epistemological challenges can arise throughout research projects. Openness to negotiate and resolve such challenges is fundamental to the capacity to create new knowledge through researching with others.

Participatory research means including different perspectives early in the process to inform fully the way in which the project is designed and carried out. Difference is actively sought to understand the varied meanings and values people attach to concepts, how they may be constructed and operationalised as research questions. This in turn leads to different methods of generating data. This approach may be regarded as more innovative in some fields than it is in others and a range of participatory practices are evident (Levac et al, 2019). But even in fields such as health and social care research where participatory research has entered the mainstream, there can still be assumptions about 'value-free' stances on the part of 'professional' researchers in contrast to evident value-based positions among those with direct experience. Everybody brings with them their evaluations of issues and experiences and these need to come into conversation as the work is carried out. This provides an opportunity for personal connections to research to be shared, and starts a conversation that can be revisited throughout the project. This was evident in a participatory research project on wellbeing in old age (Barnes et al, 2018). Growing older is an experience that is common to all, but what it means to people can be very different. The value attached to 'being old' may be rather different when one is 30 or 80. It is easy to fall into making assumptions that, for example, people do not enjoy being old. Conversations during the research were an opportunity to learn from those who were already old what good things accompany the ageing process.

What is common to effective participative ways of researching is the creation of spaces in which people are able to openly discuss ideas, with an openness to fostering and valuing difference rather than always seeking consensus. These are the spaces that we consider in more detail in Chapter 3 in which relational care can be practised. Omitting to pay attention to relationships between people in research projects can result in missed opportunities for exploration of difference, with default to academic expertise. People with experiential knowledge who contribute to research may have had little opportunity for their voices to be heard and experiences of marginalisation may be why they are part of the research in the first place. Echoing marginalisation in the research process will be felt keenly – we pick up on this point later when discussing how indigenous groups view research as a potential site of re-colonisation.

Methodology texts tend to promote a 'sink or swim' approach to research practice (see, for example, Seale, 1999, p ix). The relational skills and abilities of the researcher are second to academic skills, and managing research relationships, including the emotions that this can generate, do not really feature in such texts. But researchers need to be able to work though unpredictable situations that arise, they need both to recognise and be able to respond to the discomforts it may generate. They need to attend to preferences in how people want to be involved, and the sensitivities that may be felt in response to what is revealed through research. Emotional labour is required to work with differences in meanings and values. As in every practice, interpersonal exchanges among those working together on research require negotiation. This may need to happen quickly as well as requiring longer-term reflection. Emotional responses may generate contentious situations where immediate agreement is not possible. If we need to unsettle the fact–value, emotion–reason binaries in order to think about how to research with care, we need to look more closely at some of the contentions about knowledge and how we know, as well as address the issue of emotion more directly.

The benefits of the inclusion of direct experience in research have been clearly shown by those with positive experiences of this. One of the men Tula and Marian worked with in SureSearch went on to study for a Master's degree and then to take up a position in a university within a mental health research and development unit. Tony spoke movingly of how his involvement in carrying out research contributed to opening up new possibilities and to achieving unexpected recognition for what he could offer. There are many other such examples of beneficial impacts for those whose knowledge has been recognised and rewarded. The practical benefits of participation on the research itself are widely accepted. Brett et al (2014) have recorded a number of these. People with experience are in a better position to consider whether the research question posed is of relevance to the end user group of the research, or needs adjusting. Interview schedules may be rewritten in language that is more acceptable and accessible, and information sheets edited to be more meaningful. Users may have better strategies for recruitment and be able to critique approaches that are unrealistic or overly demanding for the target group. There may be a different prioritisation of data – so what comes out as the key message from research may alter with research results that are more relevant to the community (Wykes, 2014) and disseminated more effectively (Brett et al, 2014).

But there have also been ongoing debates about whether participation has made a real difference to the conduct of research or the knowledge this has generated. Some have questioned whether seeking to establish the impact of involvement on research is a worthwhile exercise (Beresford, 2002; Barber et al, 2012; Staddon, 2012). There has been much hope and anticipation at the possibilities of user involvement and how powerful it may be in revolutionising current practices, attitudes and service provision. The debate about how much of a revolution has occurred is ongoing – researchers tend to think that much progress has been made (Wykes, 2014) while people with experience tend to think there is much yet to be done (Simpson et al, 2014).

Alongside the practical benefits recognised by 'professional' researchers and those they invite to work with them, and the recognitional benefits experienced by those invited in as contributors, or even co-researchers, research collaborations continue to throw up problems. The most common complaint about participation is that of tokenism (Wykes, 2014): people are asked to contribute but their views are not heard, taken seriously or accepted as valid. The transformative aspirations of participatory research have often not been realised. Power and control remain with the people who extend the arm of involvement and experiences of participation are varied. Key decisions about topics, questions and methods are made outside partnership with user groups and, as Tula heard from mental health service user activists in interviews about participation in 2012, they may be excluded from discussion about priorities for change based on research findings. This means there is no opportunity to shape participation in ways that resonate with the aims of the service user movement. The emotional and physical demands on people taking part in research can be substantial (Beresford and Branfield, 2012; Bartlett, 2014) and getting to research meetings and fulfilling the tasks associated with participation can involve a considerable amount of effort. Being prepared to take on roles as research participants can mean being defined by reference to one aspect of your identity – such as that of mental health service user/survivor or an old person. Research consultant or co-worker sometimes becomes a paid role, but little attention may be paid to the challenges of reliving difficult experiences, and how this part of someone's identity determines income and employment. We are not advocating protection here, but recognition of and care for the consequences.

As people develop experience of involvement in research projects they compare those experiences and reflect on them. In a recent user involvement meeting, one woman explained how jargon was used in research group meetings. When she asked for terms to be explained, she was told that this was technical knowledge that she did not need to understand. This undermined her sense of being a valued contributor. She described feeling 'wheeled out' at public events where user involvement was cited as a positive aspect of the work, even though she had had little influence on the project.

At the same time as service users have been invited to participate in research projects because of their lived experiences, and it has been suggested that they need to have sufficiently 'worked through' their emotional responses so that they do not bring these to the work, some have also been accused of being insufficiently 'representative' precisely because of their growing experience in research. This reflects a particular type of identity dilemma (McGarry and Jasper, 2015). Researchers are interested in people because of one dimension of their identity. But, sticking with the mental health context, there are many people who have mental health problems who also work in universities or in health services (Barnes, 2015). And working with others on research projects leads (or should lead) to developing competences and the possible generation of new identities among all those taking part (see Chapter 4). The continued participation of users in research has resulted in considerable research experience alongside the experience that prompted involvement. Many users who contribute to research also have networks of action such as in non-governmental organisations, in governance positions for example as expert patients, and influence policy through those roles. These associations can help researchers leverage impact from research studies but are often an untapped source of opportunity.

Being immersed in a community and deciding to investigate that community positions researchers with an insider/outsider identity that is invaluable for multilayered understanding. But insider/outsider status also potentially creates unwanted exposure and changes relationships between the researcher and the community. We need to think about the specific dynamics and issues involved in different contexts. In the case of stigmatised identities, such as that of sex worker, some may be reluctant to risk a raised profile. How people feel about growing older may affect their preparedness to identify themselves as 'old' for the purposes of taking part as an 'older peer researcher'.

Some of the most illuminating insights into insider/outsider identities in carrying out research of this come from within indigenous communities. In the next section we consider issues relating to indigenous/non-indigenous research collaborations and their implications for researching with care in more detail.

### Indigenous knowledges

We have identified the way in which one aspect of colonialism has been to assert the supremacy of western knowledge systems and to devalue indigenous knowledge. This has significant implications for the way in which good collaboration between researchers from indigenous and non-indigenous communities can happen. Every researcher will experience this differently, but there is insufficient guidance about how to pre-empt or negotiate the inevitable repercussions from research collaborations that bring together not only people from different cultures, but that also draw on different ways of knowing. Indigenous people were creating scientific knowledge prior to the arrival of colonisers and have continued to do so since. Indigenous scientific approaches may be 'new' to academia, but are far from new in indigenous societies (McGregor et al, 2018). What has changed is that indigenous knowledge creation adopts and adapts non-indigenous knowledge into its worldview. Social research on indigenous life has, at times, failed to understand either the indigenous worldview or the existence of indigenous knowledge. It has also functioned to extract indigenous knowledge and present it to the world from the non-indigene gaze in a further act of colonisation. One result has been that indigenous communities view research as a 'dirty word' (Smith, 1999/2012). In this context it is important the researchers seek to repair the harms that have been done. As with many historical harms, there is a tendency to think that we live in post-colonial times and no longer deny the legitimacy of indigenous knowledge. But the impacts of colonisation continue to be felt every day. Non-indigenous researchers who research indigenous issues do not always do so in good partnerships with indigenous communities, nor in ways that are in solidarity with community aims.

A recent indigenous and non-indigenous research partnership project (Edwards et al, 2020; see www.indigenous.ncrm.ac.uk), funded to guide non-indigenous researchers approaching indigenous communities, identified several problems with non-indigenous approaches and suggested practices designed to enable researchers to be mindful of continuing impacts of colonisation. One issue concerned access to indigenous communities for the purpose of carrying out research. We have already noted that help in accessing mental health service users was one perceived benefit of involving service users as co-researchers. Deb McGregor discussed how indigenous communities have different criteria (than university ethics committees, for example) for whether the research should be adopted within the community. The most striking of these criteria was whether research '*shows love for future generations*' (Deb McGregor on www.indigenous.ncrm.ac.uk/resources/; emphasis added). Showing love means that the research aligns with the aims of sovereignty of indigenous communities, while acknowledging and protecting unique intellectual and ceremonial properties. It is also committed to the improvement of the conditions of life for future generations.

Indigenous research comes from a worldview that is not directly translatable into western concepts and language. This can mean quite fundamental challenges for researchers applying concepts and adopting methodologies that are 'taken for granted' in western culture. For example, there is no place in collective cultures for the 'individual', but most western research is based on the experience of the individual not the collective. While western researchers will aggregate individual responses to look for patterns of behaviour, belief or values across social groups, indigenous people responding to interview questions are likely to speak *about* the group rather than themselves as individuals. Another would be that a concept such as *whakapapa* in Te Ao Māori (Māori worldview) may loosely be translated as ancestry, but while this would be understood as direct blood lines in western cultures, it may be much broader than that for Māori. For example one *iwi* (tribe) in Aotearoa New Zealand have demonstrated the need for a river, the Whanganui, to have human rights as recognition of the living connection to the *iwi*. Including a non-human being within the frame of human rights is an expression of the interconnectedness of the human and more-than-human world and is a position that has been adopted in other contexts as a means of protecting the environment, other animals and non-human entities (Teuber, 2006). For researchers designing careful projects concerned with justice this means a need to broaden their focus on webs of care beyond the human.

Non-indigenous researchers need to demonstrate humility and be open to learning from the community, including the methodologies used to conceptualise, generate and share knowledge. McGregor et al (2018) detail many tools that support indigenous thinking and being. Researchers are called to examine the stories and ceremonies that may inform research approaches, and how the respect necessary to sustain relationships can be guaranteed. Researchers are also prompted to consider who they would consult in the case of an ethical dilemma and consider what that says about who holds knowledge about the community.

We suggest that a care-based approach to research can learn from indigenous knowledge and practices. Smith (1999/2012) has posed a number of critical questions for researchers from indigenous communities to all communities, that could guide researchers as they think about how to approach communities that may be experiencing the harms resulting from marginalisation and oppression. They reflect the starting point of care ethics in attentiveness and responsibility, and the hope that research will build solidarity to align with community aims. They include the importance of questioning why the research may be important and whether any of the proposed practices might be harmful. They ask researchers to reflect on the extent to which they are proposing the research to further their careers, how they think about accountability to the community and what they would do if they encountered aggressive or unethical practices in the course of the work. We suggest that these are critical questions that all researchers who are going to attend to research in a way that shows love for future generations could consider in order to approach research with care.

## Creative methods and accessing knowledge

Ethics of care, as a situated moral philosophy, looks to overcome the separation between philosophy, social science and their application in diverse fields of study. Sayer (2011) reaches out to philosophy in his take on social science, while from within moral philosophy Margaret Urban Walker (2007) recognises the need for dialogue with social science. As we recognise the need to be careful in the way we approach people who may have been denied the status of authoritative knowers, or whose knowledge derives from ways of thinking about the world that are different from prevailing western assumptions, we need to be creative in the way we engage with people in knowledge generation. The interaction between social science and work within the humanities, in particular philosophy, literature and other arts, helps us recognise and include different ways of storytelling and meaning making within our repertoire of participatory research practices.

The way in which people feel comfortable about telling their stories and explaining what matters to them varies. Not everyone wants to be interviewed and for those who have multiple experiences of recounting symptoms and circumstances for the purpose of professional diagnosis or assessment, a research interview can feel like another unwelcome intrusion. As researchers have attempted to work with groups who may be reluctant to engage with them, creative and novel engagement methods have evolved. This has included arts-based research with different communities that emphasises the importance of 'legacy' – a term that is preferred to 'impact' (Facer and Pahl, 2017); the use of collage-making and digital storytelling with refugee and asylum-seeking women (Vacchelli, 2018), and community theatre as a means of exploring citizenship in Nigeria (Abah and Okwori, 2005). Personal accounts presented in the form of stories have enabled people living with mental health problems to construct their own narratives that are largely unmediated by researcher frameworks (Barker et al, 1999). These ways of 'generating data' call forth a particular form of attentiveness on the part of researchers.

Hamington and Rosenow (2019) adopt a different perspective on the relationship between arts, care and research. They have explored what we can learn about care from poetry and what this means for caring knowledge. They suggest that some poetry can help us not only to learn *about care*, but also how *to* care. Its capacity to engage with the complexities and ambivalences of human responses to life and death 'can contribute to an epistemology of empathy that ultimately encourages caring behaviors' (Hamington and Rosenow, 2019, p 22). We pick up on this when we discuss the potential of careful research to build solidarity in Chapter 4.

Some of the most creative work that we think is important to learn from avoids the constraints of both disciplinary boundaries and an exclusive focus on human individuals (Tsing, 2015; Haraway, 2016). In Anna Tsing's work exploring lives lived on the margins and profoundly impacted by the devastations wrought by capitalism, the active agents in her accounts include not only human collectors and traders of mushrooms from Japan to Finland to Oregon, United States, but also the prized matsutake mushrooms that thrive in forests devastated by the destructive force of human intervention. Her work draws from and transcends anthropology, cultural studies, ecology and political economy. She deliberately plays with assumptions about divisions of labour that separate accounts of human and non-human beings, and about the 'right' way to present scholarly work. She writes:

Unlike most scholarly books, what follows is riot of short chapters. I wanted them to be like the flushes of mushrooms that come up after a rain: an over-the-top bounty; a temptation to explore; an always too many. The chapters build an open-ended assemblage, not a logical machine ... this book sketches open-ended assemblages of entangled ways of life, as these coalesce in coordination across many kinds of temporal rhythm. (Tsing, 2015, p viii)

The flawed but nevertheless important moves to increase diversity among those admitted to be part of research within the academy have supported a diversity of approaches to ways of knowing. Communities who have not previously had a chance to direct research now do so, and creative thinkers both inside and beyond the academy work together to better understand, but also to seek change, in response to the interconnected issues of human wellbeing, environmental degradation and the climate crisis. A recognition of the importance of understanding how people value and evaluate what happens to them will often require creative methods capable of tapping into more than intellectual reflections on life, and of understanding the interconnectedness and interdependencies of lived and living experiences.

As we advocate for researching done with care we are proposing methods that enable us to embrace the complications and messiness of life, that provide knowledge rich in complexities and inextricable interdependencies (Kittay, 2015). Haraway uses the image of string figures to explicate this. String figures are a form of continuous weaving practices used to tell the stories of the constellations, and of the emergence of the Navajo people. The co-making of string figures enables us to understand important things about Navajo life:

It matters which ideas we think other ideas with; my thinking or making a cat's cradle with *na'atl'o* is not an innocent universal gesture, but a risky proposition in relentless historical contingency. And these contingencies include abundant histories of conquest, resistance, recuperation, and resurgence. Telling stories together with historically situated critters is fraught with the risks and joys or composing a more livable [*sic*] cosmopolitics. (Haraway, 2016, pp 14–15)

The cultural specificity of this form of storytelling helps us know in ways not accessible through other means. It will not work in other contexts. Creating the right opportunities for people to participate in research will become apparent from within the communities themselves. Activities that people ordinarily participate in, in the groups usual for participation, will often need to be the starting point for research. In Part II we describe other ways in which familiar and unfamiliar activities can enable creative participation.

## Conclusion

In her early work on care ethics Tronto (1993) identified three moral boundaries: that between morality and politics; the 'moral point of view' boundary; and the personal is political boundary. In this work we are addressing another boundary: that of epistemology. That is a boundary not only between ways of thinking and researching, but between those who are considered authoritative knowers and who are recognised as capable of creating new knowledge, and those who are suspect both as informants and participants in knowledge generation. This is a boundary that participative research practices seek to remove. There have been important developments in this respect, but both the legacy of harms done and the absence of a sufficient focus on the relational characteristics of research practice mean we all still have much to learn. Thinking about why we research, what our relationship is to the topic of research and how that is different for others involved in these processes, is a starting point for designing and undertaking research with care. We can then focus not only on the technicalities of methodology, but also on the relationality of the research process.

# 3

# Relational research

We have seen that attempts to separate knowledge from values and objective stances from subjective engagement are impossible to sustain and that any ethical approach to research must consider what matters to people, who the research impacts and in what way. These arguments are not new – critical social scientists have been struggling with them for decades. But positivist assumptions endure, and simplistic linear models of impact continue to be used in assessing research value. Ethical procedures focus primarily if not exclusively on the capacity of researchers to predetermine ethical challenges and develop procedural mechanisms to specify how these will be met. Methodology texts prioritise techniques for data collection and analysis rather than focusing on the researcher as a practitioner engaged in creating and sustaining relationships capable of improving wellbeing and contributing to social justice objectives. This all means that it is still necessary to find ways of understanding what it means to recognise research as a dynamic, relational and political – as well as ethical – practice. What does researching with care actually mean in practice?

As we started working on this book we reflected on experiences that, as new researchers, had troubled us and suggested to us that we were somehow not getting it right, that we were failing in what it meant to be a good researcher. Often those troubles emerged out of insecurities and uncertainties concerning our relationships with those we were researching. Research encounters were often unpredictable and we felt unprepared to deal with the responses of those we approached to take part in our projects. And if we did in some way anticipate reluctance, anxiety or confrontation on the part of those we sought to research, it was not possible to specify in advance what would be the 'right' way for us as researchers to respond. Those troubles suggested we were somehow failing if we focused on the relationships generated within a research project rather than on the techniques of the particular methodology we were employing; if we mixed up emotions (ours or those of the people we were researching) with evidence, or acknowledged that our personal histories or experiences might impact our scholarship.

There are particular memories that focus some of these troubles. In my early days as a researcher, I (Marian) remember the anxieties I felt visiting people's homes to conduct interviews. I was anxious about how well I would conduct the interview and sometimes hoped the person would not answer the door so I could put off having to do the interview. One day, carrying out a study of parents caring for children with learning disabilities, the door was answered by a young woman. As she hesitantly invited me in, I realised that she was nervous of me and of what I was there to do. This was the first time I was able to recognise that others might perceive me to be in a powerful position in relation to them and that my responsibilities as a researcher meant that I needed to focus on how my actions could impact others in this context. Another experience that stands out for me occurred in a study of collective action by disabled people and mental health service users. I and my colleagues aimed to practice our research in an inclusive way by sharing interim findings with those we had interviewed in the groups we studied. When I fed back to one disabled people's group I was unprepared for the responses this generated regarding conflicts the research had exposed among activists. Members of the group had not previously confronted their own disagreements. Group members were unconcerned about the anonymity promised to other readers of the research – what bothered them was the fact that *they* recognised anonymised interviewees who were quoted and thus were confronted with internal differences that were challenging to them. And working in the mental health field we (Tula and Marian) both encountered professional responses that questioned our preparedness to believe what our respondents told us about their experiences of services. Elsewhere a senior colleague remarked to one of us that he sometimes felt the need to explain to those he interviewed for research on the topic of disability that his interest was not in the people who were recounting their experiences as people, but in the issues that their lives pointed to. At the time these were received as words of wisdom to be taken as a guide to how to approach research. Now we're not so sure. If we are arguing that we need to approach research with care, does this mean that we care about the issues but not the people or other entities we research? Is believing what people say the same as agreeing with them or assuming that this is the only way of looking at things? Does exposing differences within the groups we study matter more in terms of understanding the complexity of activism than the danger of damaging what may be quite fragile alliances? And what about the people we research with, does our relationship with our co-researchers matter and if so what does that mean for our research practice?

These are some of the questions that have troubled us as we have pursued research that we have hoped and intended to generate benefit for people who have often been marginalised and/or who are in vulnerable situations. These issues have troubled us because we care about the lives and experiences of those we research as well as the issues that are raised by them. And, while we do not assume our work will change the world, we do not want to create further harm and we do hope to make some difference. We are not alone facing these troubles. We do not presume to offer definitive answers in this book. But we do think there is a way of thinking about them that offers help to researchers who continue to confront them.

In this chapter we develop our thinking about research that embraces the importance of understanding what matters to those we research, that recognises that views from different somewheres offer a better chance of generating real understanding than a view from a single place, and that can be a way of exploring things that matter to us as people who include 'researcher' in a description of who we are. As we start to unpack what we mean by arguing that research can be a caring practice, that it is one of the things we can do that can both enable or frustrate attempts to live in the world together as well as possible, we need to consider research as a process to be undertaken with care. And this, in turn, necessitates a focus on research relationships as relationships of care. In Chapter 2 we adopted the lens of knowledge to argue for research that is democratic, inclusive and careful about the different types of knowledge people hold and how they might be shared. Here we focus more directly on the different encounters and different relationships that need to be established as we carry out research. From her reading of Haraway's work, Puig de le Bellacasa (2017, p 69) claims: 'That knowledge is situated means that knowing and thinking are unconceivable without the multitude of relations that make possible the worlds we think with.' Here we start to look at what those relations consist of in care-full research.

We start by going back to the beginning of care ethics.

## Noticing who's left out and what is not said

Carol Gilligan's book *In a Different Voice* has been published and re-published since it first appeared in 1982. One version was published in 1993 and includes an introduction in the form of a letter from the author to readers. In this Gilligan locates her writing of the original text in a time leading up to the ground-breaking *Roe v Wade* case that legalised abortion in the United States. She cited this as a ruling that awarded women the highest voice in the complex relational decision making about life and death, decisions that are emotionally and ethically challenging. She suggested that the ruling emerging from *Roe v Wade* helped women more generally to become aware of internal voices to which they had struggled to give expression, and that they had suppressed for fear of being accused of 'selfishness'. The precarity of this judgement's impact is evident from continuing campaigns in the United States to repeal *Roe v Wade*. Gilligan writes of the way in which her subsequent work as a feminist psychologist was grounded in listening and hearing what she calls the 'disconnection and dissociation' (1993, p xiii) in both men's and women's voices as they struggled with ethical dilemmas and definitions of self.

Exploring the nature and source of those disconnections, and later how and with what effect it could become possible to reconnect and resist becoming disconnected in the first place, formed the core of her work throughout her academic career (Gilligan, 2011). Gilligan described herself primarily as a woman who listens. As she listens carefully she hears ways in which we can tell false stories of our lives. These stories come from resisting what we know because this contradicts received or dominant wisdom that tells us we are either mistaken or not worthy. Fricker's (2007) work discussed in the previous chapter develops this through her notions of epistemic injustice. Gilligan's starting point in the psychology of resistance led her to a more political arena based in the recognition that 'the requisites for love and for citizenship in a democratic society are one and the same. Both voice and the desire to live in relationships inhere in our human nature, along with the capacity to resist false authority' (Gilligan, 2011, p 12).

One example of the consequences of identifying, locating and giving voice to what has been hidden comes in research Gilligan undertook in a girls' school. Her research led her to talk about what was not being spoken of as the girls struggled to negotiate the right thing to do in response to an 'honor code' they did not believe in. While they all ostensibly adhered to this code, in practice it was being subverted by girls who knew that to sustain relationships required them to manage conflict in private rather than following 'agreed procedures'. When she speaks of this as she reports research findings to teachers Gilligan records:

Silence washes over the room. The research had exposed what goes on beneath the surface. Girls' voices, recorded in private and amplified in the public space of the school, resonated with women teachers, encouraging them to ask themselves: what were they teaching girls about relationships, about speaking, about conflict, about disagreement, about psychological and political resistance? (2011, p 152)

Listening, but then vitally, enabling unheard or unexpressed voices to be heard and attended to by others, generates a recognition among those in more powerful positions that it is their practice that causes the silence. The upshot in this case was the establishment of retreats, led by members of the research team, at which the teachers could reflect on these questions and find ways of doing things differently. Following through on the findings of research created the possibility of going beyond exposing the problem and acting to repair the harms being done.

Gilligan's own work was partly a response to that of the influential psychologist Lawrence Kohlberg with whom she had worked for some time early in her academic career. Kohlberg's work had described the development of moral judgement from childhood to young adulthood.

The theoretical position he developed was based in longitudinal empirical research carried out over 20 years, from the late 1950s to the late 1970s. This research followed the development of 84 boys. It generated scales that Kohlberg argued had universal application in assessing and measuring moral development. When these scales were applied in practical situations, girls and women were frequently assessed as deficient in comparison to boys and men. Reflecting on that Gilligan wrote:

> [T]he so-called objective position which Kohlberg and others espoused within the canon of traditional social science research was blind to the particularities of voice and the inevitable constructions that constitute point of view. However well-intentioned and provisionally useful it may have been, it was based on an inerrant neutrality which concealed power and falsified knowledge. (1993, p xviii)

Neutrality can be a constraint on care. Researching in a way that reinforces silences and absences cannot generate the knowledge that comes from thinking with diverse others. In what might appear to readers today as an example of extremely restrained critique, Gilligan offers a reflection on this in the first chapter of *In a Different Voice*: 'When one begins with the study of women and derives development constructs from their lives, the outline of a moral conception different from that described by Freud, Piaget or Kohlberg begins to emerge and informs a different description of development' (1993, p 19). We, and many others, go further today. The exclusion of girls from Kohlberg's work is evidence of a failure to recognise the significance of gender in informing individual development and collective values. In Tronto's (1993) terms it fails in the first phase of what it means to care. The work is not attentive to the lives of half the population. It is not possible to attend to those who are not present in the research that claims to understand their lives. It is a moral failure in itself and is the source of multiple harms.

Encapsulated here we see the political import of an attitude that assumes that it is acceptable to base universal theories of development on research studies of one gender. It did not, apparently, matter that such theories were based on empirical research only involving 84 boys. The consequences were profound. Decisions about who should be included, or who it was convenient to include in research, determined how moral maturity is assessed. It is a short and easy route from here to assumptions about who should have a say in decisions about women's bodies and lives.

The particular insight that troubled Gilligan was that Kohlberg's theory proposed a hierarchical view of moral judgements that placed an emphasis on the application of a logical view of rights and duties as superior to moral deliberations prioritising connections and relationships. Listening to both girls and boys, women and men, as they explored moral dilemmas that they had experienced in their own lives, as well as talking through their responses to experimental vignettes, led Gilligan to distinguish the different voices that were sometimes competing with each other for expression. It was this that led to her distinction of care ethics from justice ethics in moral judgement. The implications of this are far-reaching for an understanding of the necessity of responsibility expressed in the grounding of the self in relations with others.

Listening to young people talk about the dilemmas and conflicts they experience as they try to make sense of themselves in relation to others and others' expectations of them, illuminates the sterility of a moral philosophy that avoids engaging with the messy realities of people's lives. What care ethics offers is the fundamental but profound recognition that relationality and interdependence are ontological necessities, not ideals to be aimed for through the establishment of contracts. To be human is to be in relation to others. It is through our encounters with others that we survive, are nurtured, grow and know ourselves. More than that, humanity does not and cannot sustain itself without other species and other entities. We encounter, are impacted by and have an impact on the places in which we live, the animals and plants who share those places with us, as well as the material creations of both artisanal labour and technoscience. Feminist philosophers such as Margaret Urban Walker (2007) have developed the key insight that moral and social identities and understandings are intertwined: 'Morality is woven through the way that people live; it both shapes and is shaped by the rules, roles and assumptions that constitute a social world' (p ix). Moral philosophy needs social science. And as we discussed in Chapter 2, social scientist Andrew Sayer (2011) demonstrates the absurdity of trying to exclude 'things that matter to people' from a central place in social research. Social science needs moral philosophy. As we research lives and experiences we cannot but research relationships, what they mean to people and how they bring into being identities and experiences. What gets rather less attention is the way in which research is carried out through relationships.

The world has changed a lot since the time when Kohlberg was carrying out his research. One hopes that researchers seeking funding for work intended to explore something as fundamental as human development today would get short shrift if their research design only included boys. But would we be right to make such an assumption? We know that much research with apparent broad intended application, whether it be drug testing, car safety design or decisions about office heating based on average metabolic rates, is based on assumptions that the male body can be taken as generating findings relevant to both sexes (Criado Perez, 2019). Caroline Criado Perez's review of the data biases that underpin decisions that profoundly affect the lives of us all points to a continuing invisibility of women across all fields of research.

The 'default male' endures in the 21st century. In some cases women are deliberately excluded from research because it is seen to be too messy and difficult to take account of the impact of menstrual cycles or hormones. To exclude, deliberately or otherwise, girls and women from research that is intended to draw conclusions relevant to both genders demonstrates a lack of care about women in general and about the individual women or girls who may be harmed as a result. And we extend this conclusion to other exclusions based in 'race', sexuality, age, disability and other aspects of identity that we know intersect to create very different life experiences. As we noted in Chapter 2, when one of us was confronted by a clinical psychologist arguing that we were wrong to ask people who had been compulsorily detained in a psychiatric hospital to describe the processes that led up to their admission because, by definition, they lacked insight, this not only sought to devalue the research findings we were presenting, but undermined any suggestion that people using mental health services should be regarded as having a legitimate contribution to make as to how they were provided. Assumptions that the voices of people defined in terms of a psychiatric diagnosis are suspect and thus should not be heard have become less dominant but still exist. It is not enough to argue that researchers should be alert to the exclusions they may build in to the design of research projects, but they should also be attentive to the way in which they generate diverse encounters through which knowledge is generated and change made possible.

Research is as political an activity as it is a scholarly one. What gets researched, how, and by whom reflects and reinforces power structures. We can subject research to a similar analysis to that applied by ethics of care scholars to critical policy analysis (Sevenhuijsen, 1998; Williams, 2004) and to different forms of social practice (Lloyd, 2010; Langford, 2019). Research is one of the things that we do that impacts on our capacity to live together in the world as well as possible.

As we think about how we research in future projects we need to acknowledge the way in which past research practices have caused harms that need to be repaired. We have considered the harms resulting from epistemic and cognitive injustice, and the harms resulting from the unthoughtful exclusion of half the human population from studies claiming to generate findings applicable to women and men. One particular study − of the lives of disabled people in a residential home (Miller and Gwynne, 1972) − caused outrage among disabled people because the researchers identified with staff and managers of the home and referred in their report to the inevitable 'social death' of disabled people living there. Even more shocking, there are notorious instances of the extremes to which research can go when a lack of care is based in complete disregard for the humanity of particular groups: in the United States the Tuskagee studies deliberately withheld treatment for syphilis from Black men in order to record the natural term of the disease.

The withholding of the treatment resulted in the men's deaths. The US government eventually apologised for the studies and the deaths of the men involved. The most disturbing fact about the studies was not that the treatments were withheld, but that the experiments were carried out over a very long period of time from 1932 to 1972, and that they were repeated numerous times. Black lives absolutely did not matter. The long-term harms caused by such experiences and collective memories of them is evident in the reluctance of some Black people to agree to receive vaccinations to reduce the likelihood of contracting COVID-19. Experiments on Jews and others in concentration camps resulted in the Nuremberg Code, a call for informed consent by anyone involved in research studies following numerous atrocities delivered as research projects. We return to this in Chapter 8.

It is still rather unusual to argue that researchers should expand their caring, ethical concerns to the more-than-human world. Puig de la Bellacasa (2017) emphasises the 'speculative' nature of her approach to taking care ethics into the worlds of soil biodiversity and other non-human things. But the harms done by a disregard for matters beyond the human, and by anthropocentric thinking, study and actions, should encourage us to at the very least to avoid working in ways that make invisible other entities with whom we are interconnected in webs of care. When we invited people to suggest 'what matters to us' in a consultation about an international ethics of care project, responses included the environment and climate change as a concern for the future for people's families; waste and unnecessary use of resources; and homelessness in the local community. These were a counterpoint to the issues of access to health and social care; democracy; and migration that the researchers had identified from common concerns across Europe, and helped add more detailed and real concerns to the bid.

What these very different examples illustrate is that research and researchers do not start on a level playing field with many of those they research. Research has, in some cases, been experienced as exploitative and oppressive and has become a site for challenge and contention. The Miller and Gwynne (1972) study already referred to is often cited as a key moment in the emergence of a politicised disability movement in the UK. We are not arguing that researchers should adopt uncritical perspectives in the work they do and automatically assume that the positions advocated by those they research are the only way of looking at things. But we are arguing that they should be attentive to previous harms resulting from failures to recognise the operation of unequal power; to the relationships they build through their own research, and the danger that these unequal power structures will be reproduced with future consequences of their work for those who are already marginalised. In a recent 'letter from the editor', Derek Clifford, long-standing joint editor of *Ethics and Social Welfare*, appealed for a more political ethical awareness in research: 'My contention is that mainstream research in much healthcare in the UK (and elsewhere) *tends to avoid* difficult yet crucial issues of social division and social structure that play out in the micro-social world of research ethics' (Clifford, 2019, p 434; original emphasis). If we are to stop avoiding these difficult issues we need to focus on who's who within the research process and on the relational aspects of doing research.

## Relating to research

We discussed in Chapter 2 how Andrew Sayer (2011) elegantly reminds us that we are social beings for whom things matter. We evaluate things and make assessments of what is important to us. To try to bracket out the evaluative, subjective and normative from our analysis of the behaviour, capacities, experiences, ideas, suffering and vulnerabilities of those we study as social scientists is an absurdity. But so too is it to pretend that we researchers into the lives of those we share the planet with can avoid our own nature as social beings with our own interdependencies and vulnerabilities. How we practice relationality within research brings our own selves into dialogue with others.

Let us pick up on our argument that we do research on topics that matter to us, that we care about. Why else would we spend our time and energy focusing in depth on any particular topic? Let us leave to one side the purely financial issue of a necessity for paid employment – there are other choices to be made if the motivation is solely about generating an income. Some, most, of those who 'do research' do this as all or part of a job – as an academic, in a policy research institute, or in an applied field (medicine or IT, say) where development is predicated on generating new knowledge and understanding. Research students undertaking doctoral research are not, except in limited circumstances, employed to carry out the research they do. In advising potential research students Marian often reminded them that this might be the only time in their research career that they were virtually free to choose what they want to research because it is not linked to some aspects of an employment contract. But they are usually either embarking on a career that will continue to include research as a significant part of their work, or they are employed in organisations that recognise research as either/both integral to professional development or/and the development of the work of that organisation. In these contexts there are varying degrees of choice regarding the topic of research and these intersect with varying degrees of frustration (or worse) regarding the tension between what is necessary for career development and what personal interests, commitments and values might lead you towards. Sometimes caring about an issue may mean being subversive in the way in which it can be approached (Barnes and Prior, 2009) and applying for research funding can include considerable skill in responding effectively to funders' criteria while also remaining true to personal and political values.

But the key point we want to make here is that the relationship of those undertaking research as part of their job to the topic being studied can be very different from the relationship that others who are also involved in or affected by research have to this. The same topic often matters in very different ways to people who are differently positioned in the research process. They may all care about the issue, but for some it may be, literally, a matter of life or death; it may speak to difficult or distressing aspects of their everyday lives, and it may undermine or strengthen an aspect of their identity that is important to them. A researcher who does not directly share such experiences (neither of us has ever been admitted to a psychiatric hospital for example, although we have both researched with those for whom this has been a significant part of their lives) cannot know from personal experience what this feels like, although they can care about its consequences for others. A different position in relation to the topic goes beyond having different views about it. We can offer examples to illustrate what we mean before going on to explore some of the implications from an ethic of care perspective. The following examples draw on our own experiences and thus emphasise applied research in a health and social care context.

Evaluations of services or policies can feel very threatening to practitioners who think that they are being judged by researchers who know less about the work than they do and who do not have to negotiate the everyday realities of practice. Reassurance that evaluative critique is about exposing the limitations of policies, the inadequacy of resourcing, or the value of learning in order to do better, can be unconvincing when practitioners feel they are being exposed to criticism for failures either of process or outcome. But there are different ways of undertaking evaluations that can mitigate a sense of being judged. One such approach, designed initially to offer a way of evaluating complex community initiatives, is theories of change evaluation (Connell et al, 1995). In this approach, rather than working to a set of predetermined outcome indicators, evaluators work with groups directly involved in the initiative to surface their theories of change and then use these as a framework within which to assess whether and how well the programme is achieving what initiators hoped to achieve. This approach originated in work undertaken by researchers in the United States involved in community development programmes working with and for children and families. It was not only a response to the inadequacies of randomised controlled trial models of evaluation in such contexts, but was also designed to recognise both the different relationships different groups had to the programme and the likelihood that learning and improvement would be strengthened by involvement in the process of evaluation. It was subsequently applied in evaluations of what became known as 'complex community initiatives' in the UK, such as the Children's Fund – a national, government-funded programme designed to address social exclusion by working with families and young children (Morris et al, 2009), and Health Action Zones, established to address both health inequalities and the need for health improvement in the most deprived areas of England (Barnes et al, 2005).

In theory of change evaluation not only are programme participants recognised as thoughtful contributors to programme design and implementation, but also as collaborators in the design of the evaluation. Researchers need to reflect on their roles and their relationships to those whose work and projects they are evaluating. The processes by which those relationships are established are not only crucial to determining the research focus, but also enable learning and development in their own right. Such processes can surface disagreements and conflict as well as enable shared articulations and assumptions (Brown, 1998; Mason and Barnes, 2007). What evaluators are able to do is not only to assess the extent to which objectives have been achieved, but if things have not worked out as anticipated, why that was the case. The relationship between researchers and programme participants is thus very different from in traditional evaluation approaches. Both are involved in a process that seeks to learn from what goes wrong as well as what works. While the word 'care' may not appear in the theories of change literature, it is evident from the start that the researchers must care not only about the programme, but also about those directly involved in it if they are to work effectively to carry out the evaluation. A more explicitly care ethical approach to evaluation is the responsive evaluation described by Visse and her colleagues (Visse et al, 2015). Here the roles played by researchers extended to that of advocate and dialogue facilitator in the context of a multi-agency project experiencing unsurfaced differences between professionals with different professional backgrounds. By focusing on 'responsibilities' as understood within care ethics, the evaluators sought to support a learning process among participants intended to enable 'good care'.

We discussed in Chapter 2 the way in which research became both a site for contention and a means for pursuing social justice projects and campaigning for improved services among disabled people, mental health advocacy groups and other users of health and social care services (Sweeney et al, 2009; Barnes and Cotterell, 2012). At the same time, collective action on the part of disabled people and others using health and welfare services has become a subject for research attention in its own right (Barnes et al, 1999). We referred at the start of this chapter to a difficult encounter when feeding back interim findings to a disabled people's group. Mental health activists involved in self-advocacy and campaigning projects can feel that their project is being reinterpreted or even taken over by academic researchers of social movements and their own analysis and interpretation of events is hidden behind the profile and theoretical preferences of the researcher. One of the consequences of collective action by survivors has been to recognise the importance of telling their own stories and recounting their own histories.[1] This can lead to distress when others tell the story in different ways. At a conference organised by Marian one speaker was an academic researcher of social movements who had published a book on the mental health user/ survivor movement. When she invited him, Marian had not realised that this research had caused anger among some activists concerned at aspects of the way in which the research had been carried out and some of the interpretations offered. The speaker (and Marian as Chair of the conference session) was confronted by angry responses by activists present that challenged the academic's authority to speak on their behalf and threatened to disrupt the session. The emotion that can be generated by research broke out and demanded an immediate response. Marian found this hard to deal with in the moment, but communications with the man who had led the challenge after the event achieved some resolution and enabled better understanding of the reasons for the response.

The general point we want to make is that 'caring about' as a starting point for research not only reveals what matters to us, but also is the starting point for the way in which we approach the practice of research and the relationships we seek to develop as we go about this. We might 'care about' an issue, but that care is not always evident to those we encounter as we establish the different relationships necessary to carry out the research we do and as we seek to disseminate our own work and that of others. In some instances the fact that researchers care about an issue might be experienced as appropriating it – Marian was accused of trying to 'take over' the survivor movement in the challenge reported in the previous paragraph. The people we research may not feel cared for, nor are they able to demonstrate their capacity to give care in the process of the research being done. They may feel 'done to' by the research in a way that is similar to their experience of being 'cared for'. Both leave disabled people and survivors feeling powerless to shape their own lives (Campbell and Oliver, 1996). One response has been to seek to take control of the research process in a way comparable with the objective of taking control over personal support. And that, in some cases, meant arguing for, for example, disability research to be conducted only by disabled people (Barnes and Mercer, 1997).

We absolutely support that people with experience lead research, and are encouraged by the initiatives that promote capacity building and leadership in this sector. But we don't think this is the only way. What we are proposing is 'researching with' people directly affected by the topic of research. And we are arguing that to research with people necessitates researching with care. In her response to Donna Haraway's work Puig de la Bellacasa (2017) explores the necessity of 'thinking with care' in her speculation on ethics in more-than-human worlds. She suggests that thinking with care invites a 'thinking-with committed to a collective of knowledge makers, however loose its boundaries and complex its shapes' (p 75). We want to offer some shape to those collectives without defining boundaries that might constrain how they operate. The contextual nature of care *and* research mean that blueprints can lead to unhelpfully narrow designs that will not work in all circumstances. Some of the examples we consider in this book do not involve the active involvement of 'research subjects' in the process of doing research, but many of them do. Because of the histories and encounters that we have outlined in this and the previous chapter, for us researching in the fields that we do, research as a practice of care does need to find ways of enabling those whose lives are the subject of research to be active subjects in the doing of research. So it is this that we will prioritise in the stories we tell. Tula's research in partnership with Māori adopted an ally approach that acknowledged and appreciated what the ethics of care could learn from Kaupapa Māori. This was an emphasis on relational care in everything that is done, the framing of the issue in its position to colonisation, and the presence of the past, present and future in all thinking (Boulton and Brannelly, 2015; Brannelly and Boulton, 2017).

## Who is involved in research?

At this point it is helpful to spell out the different types of people who are likely to be involved in research projects, but who have different relationships with the research process. Research is as varied a practice as the contexts within which it takes place. Our perspective, that starts from the research worlds that we are most familiar with from our work in health and public services, offers particular insights into the diverse participants in the research process and may be rather different from that experienced by, for example, those working in the fields of moral philosophy or even sociology. We have been stimulated by the work of those taking post-disciplinary approaches to research (such as Donna Haraway and Anna Tsing) and we hope it is helpful to think about the different relationships to research that our starting point in care ethics suggests, regardless of the discipline of each researcher or the field in which they practice.

Books about research do not often consider those who fund and also possibly commission research in terms of their relationships to it. That includes bodies dedicated solely to research funding, such as UK research councils, but, in our world, also national and local governments, health service commissioners and providers, non-governmental organisations, commercial agencies and other bodies seeking to base policies, practices or services on research evidence. Commissioning research could be understood as one way of evidencing care for an issue. A problem or need is identified as requiring attention, better knowledge and understanding is seen to be necessary in order to determine what action is needed, resources are allocated and competent 'experts' sought to carry out research to inform policy and practice. In times of obvious need or crisis, research evidence becomes recognised as a key resource for policy making that can generate most benefit: the COVID-19 pandemic is a contemporary example of this; the ongoing impact of climate change is another. Both examples demonstrate both the degree to which researchers are motivated by their care for the issue they are researching, and the sometimes problematic relationship between this care and what it is that policy makers care about. Experience demonstrates that to think of the process of commissioning research as 'caring' about the problem or need being explored is not always a warranted assumption. Personal experience of conducting government-funded evaluations where policies have changed before the research is complete – as in the Health Action Zones project referred to earlier – or of reporting findings only to be told that stated programme objectives no longer apply so the premise on which the research was based are not relevant, indicate other motivations can drive research commissioning. And the relationship between commissioners and those who carry out the research during the course of the project may be unlikely to attract a description as a relationship of care.

Nevertheless, we should consider not only how the way in which research is commissioned and funded impacts on the capacity of researchers to carry out their work with care, but also the possibility that commissioners and funders can be included in a web of care in which research is an important contributor to beneficial policy and practice development. The work of Connelly and his colleagues (2017) is one example of ways in which research and policy communities can work together to develop alliances and better understanding. This was part of a broader programme of work in which the idea of 'impact' was transformed to that of 'legacy': 'we need a language for talking about new models of change, in which there is a recognition that the legacies of these projects might emerge in tangential or unexpected ways' (Pahl and Facer, 2017, p 221). These examples illustrate possibilities grounded in diverse enactments of shared care for the people and issues at stake.

Tula had a personal experience of research commissioners being attentive to the relational ethics of research practice. She had a panel interview for a service evaluation grant in Wellington, Aotearoa New Zealand. There were two services involved, one of which was Kaupapa Māori – or run by and for Māori, and the team was a partnership between Māori and Pākehā researchers. At the interview, the panel asked how a British woman was going to ensure that the people who contributed to the project did not feel colonised, and whether there was an awareness of the prospect for colonialism in the project. Although initially confronting, as Tula is Irish, this was a welcome question that enabled a discussion about how best to deliver the project in a way that enabled the partnership to conduct the research in the best way possible.

While lone research is possible research projects often require a team to carry them out. Members of that team may have specific roles associated with particular skill sets or seniority. Those undertaking research interviews or other types of data collection may not have been involved in project design and specialist expertise may be required for statistical analysis, or negotiating access to groups that may be reluctant to take part. One or more senior team members are likely to have responsibilities related to financial management and project administration that can seem to be very little to do with 'research', but which are essential to the effective conduct of what are often complex projects. Teams can be large or small: we have experience of working with only one or two colleagues and also of teams of up to 30 distributed across three different universities (such as the Children's Fund evaluation referred to earlier). International collaborations introduce further complexities in terms of how to sustain good working relationships. These can be particularly sensitive when those collaborations involve researchers from the global north researching with colleagues from the global south who have much more limited resources and who have experienced colonialism in the form of epistemological power (we reflect on examples of that in Part II of this book). We need to think not only about the varying relationships team members may have with the topic being researched, but also relationships within the research team. Do people feel cared for as they work together? How is caring for those carrying out the work prioritised in relation to meeting deadlines?

There are then the research participants, the people who are the 'sample', who are a key source of data that is generated. They may be all those who are a part of the study topic (for example, if the research is looking at cultures of practice on a hospital ward the researchers may observe and talk to all those currently working on the ward, as well as those who are currently patients), but more often they will have been selected and invited to take part in order to 'represent' a wider population. One difficult issue in research that involves sampling or some other form of selection is that the key characteristic that leads to selection, such as a diagnosis of dementia or experience of compulsory detention under the Mental Health Act, is only one of a number of factors that impact on the way people think about what matters to them. In both cases, that of total population or sample group, the people involved are likely to have a direct interest in the topic of the research. They may well care very much about it, but other aspects of their lives might affect the extent to which they feel cared for in the way in which the research is carried out. Tula had the experience of bringing together a group of people diagnosed with dementia for a residential research workshop. The group included people from very different backgrounds, who responded very differently to the proposal, which led to a rethink to ensure participants felt properly cared for. The intersectional nature of encounters through the research process will impact research relationships. Care-full research may seek to build solidarity among researchers and research subjects/participants, but a number of factors may impact this.

Beyond the direct participants there is the total population from which the sample is drawn or is the basis on which invitations to take part are made. Often it would be virtually impossible to identify or contact all these people directly, there are simply too many. The fluidity of identities and unhelpfulness of categorical boundaries also makes it hard to decide who might be included: for example, if we are researching the experience of growing older at what point in the life cycle should we start? Nevertheless we need to consider that the issue of ageing well is likely to matter to those who are not yet old as well as those who indubitably are. How do researchers include this wide and disparate group within their sphere of care? More fundamentally, who is making the decision about how to define who should be involved and what are the consequences of this? There is a long tradition of research on 'deprived' communities and on those who can be defined by reference to their use of welfare services. Does this in itself mean the people involved are only seen to be of interest because of their client status, vulnerability or powerlessness? We know of contexts in which people living in what are seen to be 'deprived communities' become fed up of researchers frequently seeking access – and becoming very knowledgeable about research processes as a result of being 'over researched'. And what are the consequences of limiting the study of the rich and powerful?

Then there are those who may think the topic of a research project is nothing to do with them, they don't care, for example, whether the current welfare regime leads to additional struggle and suffering for those with learning disabilities, they resist any notion that they will one day be old. To what extent do we want to persuade them that they should care about research that identifies an increase in suicide and self-harm consequent on changes in benefits rules, or which recognises old people as worthy of attention? They may have minimal relationship with research, but we may want to convince them that it should matter to them. One of the consequences of the COVID-19 pandemic has been to generate rather more interest in epidemiology than has existed before, showing that people's relationships to both issues and the research that can inform how we respond to them can change.

An important group who intersect with one or more of those we have already considered is those we can think of as users of the research. In some cases funders or commissioners are the primary users, but co-researchers also involved in campaigning around issues of disability, mental health or the needs of migrant women are also likely to have direct interests in making use of the research to support their campaigns. In other cases researchers may be seeking to influence people who have had no previous contact with the research: the researchers looking at what is necessary to counteract the soil exhaustion resulting from exploitative forms of agriculture that Puig de la Bellacasa (2017) cites are likely to seek an audience among farmers who may not have known of the projects they have been conducting. Thinking about people who we want to take note of our research as people we have a relationship with and as people who have a relationship with the research, encourages us to embrace them within an expanding network of connections that can require different types of communicative practices. The approach of all those involved will be framed by the different context of their lives and work. Establishing effective communication and understanding in order to achieve a positive legacy requires both understanding the different contexts and domains with which research findings will need to interact, and being open to the reciprocity that caring entails.

We will return to some of these questions as we develop our more detailed analysis of research practices in the next chapter and in our discussion of particular projects later in this book. But a key point that is a thread running through all our discussions is the need to recognise the relational implications of such questions. And, linked to this, is to ask and be aware of the extent to which the different groups we have distinguished in this analysis intersect and what are the implications of this.

## Conclusion

In this chapter we have considered who's who in research, who has been missing from research and why it is important to think about research relationally. As we establish relationships with the different people who are involved, we engage with the different ways in which people come to be seen as credible knowers, or not; we come face to face with the emotional responses of people to the topics we are researching, and we encounter the consequences of different degrees and types of power associated with the different positions of those who are part of the research process.

In Chapters 2 and 3 we have argued that it is important not only to ensure that the different voices of beings, human and otherwise, are heard in the research process, but also that being directly involved in doing research has made a significant contribution to achieving recognition on the part of many marginalised and excluded peoples. Others have promoted and discussed the value of co-production in research (for example Facer and Pahl, 2017; Banks et al, 2018) and some have promoted the distinctiveness of survivor research and argued for radical changes in who controls the research process if emancipatory objectives are to be achieved (Barnes and Mercer, 1997; Sweeney et al, 2009).

We do not argue that only disabled people can research experiences of disability, that non-indigenous researchers should steer clear of seeking to understand better the impacts of colonialism, or that until you are old it is pointless trying to research what contributes to wellbeing in old age. Not only does the messiness of intersectional identities mean that we are in danger of retreating into an ever-contracting spiral of limitations in determining who is allowed to research what, restricting authority to research to those sharing characteristics of experiences with 'research subjects' constrains the development of imaginative understanding and of care. Not only is it important to disrupt the damaging categorical boundaries between, for example, those diagnosed as 'mentally ill' and 'normal' human people, we also need to look to research to provide encounters that can be a way of generating care and solidarity between people and entities differently positioned in terms of power, vulnerability, injustice and marginalisation.

Donna Haraway (2016) offers imaginative leaps in which future humans embrace aspects of the being of butterflies and these interspecies learn to live in symbiosis with the non-human world in order to repair the damage done through extinctions, exterminations and genocides. How damaging, then, to think that no one who has not received a diagnosis of mental illness can try to understand through research ways in which those who have been so diagnosed have sought to resist what such a diagnosis means for the way they are viewed by others. If we can only care about those issues that relate to one aspect of our identity living well together in difference becomes impossible.

Our starting point within care ethics means that we offer a rather different perspective on participatory or co-produced research than that of many other advocates of this way of working. We need to think carefully about how we research with others and what kinds of relationships we need to establish if such collaborations are to contribute to the justice and wellbeing objectives claimed for them. It is here where we think that the relational ontology of care ethics and its capacity to make connections between the interpersonal and the political offers a valuable way of developing both our thinking and practice. We explore this in more detail in the next chapter.

# 4

# Stages of research, phases of care

Up to this point we have argued that care is a motivator for research, and we have suggested that different participants in the research process are likely to care about the topic in different ways and be differently positioned in relation to it. We have argued that generating knowledge is a relational process and that the emotional dimensions of doing research are not a messy distraction, but the source of important understandings. But we have rather skirted around what we mean by 'care-full research' in practice. In this chapter we discuss what doing research with care means in terms of the design, conduct and use of research. We link the stages of research with the phases of care articulated by Tronto (1993) in her book *Moral Boundaries* and developed in her later work (2013).

To introduce this discussion, we offer an example that comes from a world that is much less familiar to us than many of the examples we have drawn on from our own experiences as researchers. As we were discussing this book and talked of the need to go beyond the human in our consideration of doing research with care in a world in which the damage done to the biosphere and the physical environment by humans has become all too obvious, we were unsure what this might mean for the type of participatory research practice that we are advocating. Our advocacy of co-production is based on our experience of researching in a health and social care context in which research has become one strategy for pursuing social justice. We felt reasonably confident about proposing what careful participatory research means in these contexts. But is it possible to imagine research practices in which different species as well as different humans might care about an issue and collaborate and research together with care for their collective benefit? We found one answer in Donna Haraway's (2016) story of the PigeonBlog.

The 'matter of concern' that prompted this story was air pollution and how this might be measured and communicated to the people affected by it. This is a matter of concern not only to humans but also to the animals and plants who also have to breathe and try to live within polluted air. The researchers came up with an answer that not only involved collaboration among humans with different skills and knowledge, but also with pigeons who became data collectors and communicators. Racing pigeons, raised and trained by pigeon fanciers, were equipped with monitoring devices capable not only of collecting real-time data on pollution levels, but also of streaming this to the public via the Internet. Haraway describes what was involved in this cross-species collaboration in order to carry out the project in a caring and response-able way:

> The researcher-artists-engineers took about three months to design the basic technology, but making the pack small, comfortable and safe enough for the pigeons took almost a year of building hands-on multispecies trust and knowledge essential to joining the birds, technology and people. No-one wanted an overloaded homing pigeon plucked from the air by an opportunist falcon that was not a member of the project! Nobody, least of all the men who bred, raised, handled and loved their racing pigeons, would tolerate anxious and unhappy birds lumbering home under duress. The artist-researchers and pigeon fanciers had to render each other capable of mutual trust so that they could ask the birds for their confidence and skill. (Haraway, 2016, p 22)

So yes, researching with other-than-humans *is* possible in a way that is based in care and trust rather than exploitation. It is not just that we need to encompass interconnections across species and between people, places and things as we think about *what* we should research, but that *how* we do this can be enriched by recognising other species and other entities as potential contributors to the research process. We should think of them as participants and collaborators rather than things we can exploit for our own ends. Doing research with other species can encourage cross-species care. Our sense that we can learn from researchers other than social scientists about ways of researching that embody care ethics is reinforced. The people we need to collaborate with as we develop care ethical research will often be people whose skills and understanding may be in different areas of human activity, whether technological, artistic, environmental or other areas of knowledge and expertise. For example, a new funded network that Tula is a member of explores how multispecies dementia research can be developed – that brings together animals, nature and people with dementia to consider how wellbeing can be supported.[1]

We can identify a number of examples where matters of concern are not only matters of human interdependency, but of human and non-human interdependency in a world where injustices accrue to different species and where not only wellbeing but survival requires us to care about the more-than-human world. In Chapter 2 we noted the river Whanganui that has been conferred human status and protection under the Human Rights Act in Aotearoa New Zealand. The protection of sacred spaces may be with reference to a legendary being, such as a *taniwha* (supernatural creature) who may not be disturbed by the development of a road or bridge or tunnel. A relational, careful way of doing research carries the possibility not only of building solidarity through encountering and doing things together, it also enables an imaginative engagement with the lives of other beings. The learning that is possible is not only cognitive, but creative and emotional, and holds the potential for transformation as we work with others whose lives might be very different from our own.

## Research as care

So what does it mean to include research among those activities that can be considered to comprise 'care'? Certainly research is not what most people would think of in this context. But then neither would most people consider the practice of politics as an activity that can and indeed should embody care. Political care ethics shakes off the constraints of categorical boundaries that support privileged irresponsibility on the part of those who claim care is nothing to do with them. Politics itself has been subject to analysis by care ethicists (for example Mackay, 2001) and the practice of deliberative democracy has been seen to be most effective if it is done with care (Barnes, 2008, 2019b).

We have argued that 'caring about' issues, things that matters to people, in Andrew Sayer's formulation, can provide the motivation to do research. Curiosity about others, care and concern about injustices, people, issues, things that matter to us can prompt us to want to do research – both to better understand, but also to try to make a difference. 'Thinking with' necessitates recognition of the interconnectedness of those researching and those who are otherwise involved in the research process. All are, in different ways, participants in generating knowledge. But researching is not only a question of 'thinking', but of 'doing' with others. This does not necessarily mean agreement, an absence of dissent, among those whose relationships to the issue being studied may be quite different. It does not dissolve difference or resolve power differentials. But it does necessitate a willingness to open up to the possibilities of both thinking and doing together in a shared project that has the potential to have a benign and even transformative impact. And this necessitates the integrity of care-full research practices that reflect Tronto's (2013) five phases of care.

We start our development of what this means, as so often is the case, with Fisher and Tronto's definition of care (cited in Tronto, 1993, p 103). That definition opens, not with a list of activities or personal characteristics that comprise care, but with an indication that caring comprises a broad range of activities that share a common purpose. Care is *purposeful*. It seeks maintenance, continuation and repair in order to enable us to live as well as possible in the world. And here we have argued that we should expand this to emphasise the necessity of connection – care is necessary so that we can live in the world as well as possible *together*. This definition of care acknowledges that there are things that are wrong – we need not only to continue and maintain what helps us to live well, but to repair those things that have gone wrong or have never been right. Hence it seeks change and, as we and others have argued, it seeks a more fundamental project of transformation (Barnes et al, 2015). The 'why' in terms of why do research, is not only that we care about the topic in terms of having an interest in, but also in terms of wanting to do something about it, to make a difference, to repair what is broken and in doing so create something better.

Care encompasses multiple interconnected subjects. We are woven together in webs, we both give and receive care within networks that can both support and frustrate the integrity of care. Although in many applications of care ethics, as well as care practices developed from rather different starting points, both the subject of care and the care giver are individuals, Fisher and Tronto's definition speaks to the necessity of the embodied self in relation to others, and also to the environment in which they live. That environment is one of multiple encounters. It is peopled with others with whom we have intimate, distant or stranger relationships; it is structured politically and organisationally; given meaning through cultural, religious and artistic expression, and it encompasses technologies, beloved objects, other animals, plants, soil and landscapes. The maintenance, continuation and repair of all these things that are necessary to the sustenance of life in turn requires embracing them within webs of care. That applies whether we are thinking about the importance of the home environment to old people for whom it carries nurturing memory and familiar comforts, or the forests that both sustain biodiversity and absorb the carbon dioxide that is overheating our planet.

We can think of research, at the very least, as one technology that is implicated in often unknown ways in affecting the way we and others can live. But as we have indicated in our discussions up to now, research cannot be separated out from other processes named here. The knowledge making associated with research is made with and through the relationships within which it is conducted. It is now time to look more closely at what doing research with care means.

## Phases of care

### Attentiveness

Tronto's starting point for care, caring about, requires noticing, being attentive to, an issue of concern or need. It is often the case that research is focused on things that are not right, that have either gone wrong, or where it is thought that they could be improved. So who is doing the noticing, who is naming the need and framing the matter of concern? From what perspective are they looking and over what timescale are they giving attention to enable them to recognise changes that might indicate that something is wrong? Who is deciding on the scope of research programmes and making decisions about what projects should be funded? Mental health services might be operating in the correct manner according to clinicians or managers of health services, but from the point of view of those using the services all sorts of problems may be evident. Those who have a long-term relationship with a service may notice deteriorations in conditions that are not evident to a professional moving from one setting to another. Attentiveness is more than a one-off noticing, a capacity to be attentive requires a getting to know, an alertness to the meaning of behaviours and responses, an awareness of change.

Are service users able to have a say in determining priorities for research? And if they are, are they also able to frame the need, to name what requires repair, so that the research is designed in a way capable of understanding this? An increase in diagnosed mental health problems among children and young people may be a cause for concern within society generally as well as for those whose lives are blighted by mental health challenges, but who gets to define the way in which this should be researched to understand what is causing this and what might help to reduce such problems? Do we enable children to frame the problem as they see it (Brady et al, 2012)? Care starts with attentiveness, but also, we suggest, with acceptance: acceptance that the other, who may be marginalised, stigmatised or muted, is of equal worth and equally capable of knowing what is in need of repair. In Chapter 2 we discussed one dimension of (in)justice that has variously been named as 'cognitive justice' (Visvanathan, 2005) or 'epistemic (in)justice' (Fricker, 2007). Starting to do research with care requires us to acknowledge that we need to listen and to talk to others who know about things in a different way before determining the focus and scope of projects.

Thus, doing research with care necessitates attentiveness both in identifying topics and negotiating these with others involved in, impacted by, or concerned about what is to be researched. Often this can be achieved by listening and through conversation. In other cases observation and learning to understand the significance of behaviours or other non-verbal communications is necessary. In her focus on the necessity for 'attentive listening' as fundamental to social justice, Bourgault (2016) argues that listening is an embodied act requiring 'corporeal presence' (p 316) during which not only is the listener aware of facial and bodily gestures and responses of the speaker, but the speaker becomes aware of and responds to the bodily signals of the listener. And it can be the case that 'being or working alongside' creates a context of embodied presence within which the attentiveness necessary for care can start (Barnes, 2019b). Not everyone has a facility with words and it is not only across linguistic differences that we need to be careful that we have understood meanings. And even when we share the same language the significance of words and actions may not be immediately obvious. We need to take time to be properly attentive. Things that do not fit the frame at one point may subsequently be recognised as key to opening up new ideas, new ways of thinking that are necessary if we want to move beyond the limitations of received wisdom. We can offer one example here.

In the early 1990s Marian was researching collective action among disabled people and users of mental health services. One of the mental health advocacy groups involved, the Nottingham Advocacy Group (NAG), was initially established to give a voice to those in psychiatric hospitals targeted for closure in the move towards community care. Over time it evolved to provide self and collective advocacy for users of diverse mental health services. But one aspect of its work was rather different. Brian Davey, a member of the group, set up a project he called 'Ecoworks'. The focus of this project was an allotment in a deprived part of inner-city Nottingham where both users of mental health services and people living in the area could grow vegetables, meet to talk and cook meals using the vegetables they had grown. It served to enable those with psychiatric diagnoses to engage in a valuable activity; to enable both service users and local people to meet together across the barriers that separated those with and without diagnoses; it offered an opportunity to produce food cheaply for those living in poverty; it was an example of producing food in an environmentally sustainable way; and it offered a model of community development from the ground up. It was not focused on relationships between service users and the mental health system, but on their relationships with each other, with other local people and with the environment in which they lived. All of those things were implicated in their experiences of mental distress and capable of helping to repair the damage they had experienced. But others involved in NAG regarded Ecoworks as a bit of a side show. It was Brian's project, treated with a degree of condescension and marginal to the main purpose of influencing the mental health system through individual and collective advocacy. From the perspective of me and my colleagues undertaking the research it was an interesting development, but did not enable us to pursue in any detail our primary interest in the interaction between user self-organisation and professional mental health services. I visited the allotment and talked to those who were there at the time, I interviewed Brian and read with interest things that he had written, some of which were published (for example Davey, 1994), but the predetermined focus of the research did not allow me to include this as anything beyond an example of the diversity of user/ survivor activism.

The broader challenges the project faced are illustrated in a spoof paper written to indicate what would be required to enable Ecoworks to 'fit' the demands funding agencies were making on community-based projects seeking sustainable incomes:

> The Ecoworks Digitally Standard Regenerated Humans Project has been designed to embody the latest Regeneration thinking after the introduction of the General Agreement in Trade in Services. Everything in the project has been standardised into predictable standard packages of measurable products. The products chosen for measurable improvements in performance are:
>
> Carrot production
> Cabbages
> Output of composting toilet
> Lengths of paths
> Hedge heights
> The Human Resource Units.
> (Email dated 24 March 2002, personal communication)

Today Ecoworks would not be regarded as particularly radical. The insights it sought to enact through the allotment project and others that developed with similar aims of linking environmental sustainability, community development and peer support for people living with mental health problems, are much more mainstream. I regret that I and my colleagues were not sufficiently attentive to the way this group of service users had applied their knowledge of factors contributing to mental distress to offer a response that was very different from what was available from mental health professionals. We did not adapt our research design and include a more careful consideration of the role it was playing and the deliberate decision to remain separate from professional mental health services. Brian Davey expressed the need for attentiveness from service providers: 'Because the psychiatrist cannot be wrong they don't listen, and if they don't listen they complete the disempowerment of the patient and thereby render all recovery impossible' (Davey, 1994, p 131).

This applies equally to researchers. Developing appropriate skills of attentiveness is important for researchers working in all areas, but is particularly important in the context of research with people who have been disempowered, rendered speechless or considered incapable of having anything worthwhile to say. Without being attentive to those living with mental distress in the ways in which research topics are defined, researchers are in danger of reproducing the epistemic injustice elaborated by Fricker and discussed in the previous chapter. It is also vital in research with people whose methods of communications may not involve voice in any recognisable way, or whose ways of life are based in very different cultural assumptions and knowledge systems. One of the ways in which Māori practice differently is the setting of a new path for the future through a ceremony that seeks to establish connections between people (see Brannelly et al, 2013a). In relation to research, this means envisaging new possibilities for the future, new ways of doing and new relationships that will come about through the research. It is, literally, an opening. This proves an exciting prospect as change is reassuringly guaranteed, but in a way that is already considered and is dependent on engaging with diverse knowledges from the start.

In a very different context, until recently few would have thought that it is possible to enable people with dementia or those who have memory problems deriving from different causes to contribute to decisions about research topics and design. But caring enough about including people within research has led to recognition that good research practice means an attentiveness that requires repeated discussions and the collection of a number of responses that can build a picture of what people want to contribute. Repeated discussion can overcome the cognitive load that challenges people to respond (Brannelly and Bartlett, 2020). This is but one context in which attentive listening requires an unhurried approach (Bourgault, 2016).

Attentiveness goes beyond a superficial noticing. To form the basis of well-formulated research questions or design it must include thoughtfulness and a willingness to explore the potential implications of what might seem odd or surprising comments as well as the broader significance of what might appear anecdotal reflections. It requires time to get to know people and for effective communication to develop. To be attentive is not a one-off task to be completed, but requires an ongoing relationship and openness to learning and reflection.

Caring about continues throughout the research process. Attentiveness to the way in which the research is progressing may mean adjustments to the precise focus or methods being used become necessary. Attentiveness is necessary both to the topic and to the people, or other entities, involved in the research. If we had been more attentive to Brian Davey and his colleagues on the allotment in Nottingham what would this have meant for the way in which we included carrot production and the output of compostable toilets as matters of concern necessary to understanding the empowerment of mental health service users? Although it would have required an adjustment to our research questions part way through the project, we may have been able to make a more substantial, early contribution to understanding the relationship between the natural environment, individual wellbeing and collective empowerment than we were in a position to do.

## Responsibility

The second phase of care is 'taking care of' – accepting the responsibility to act in response to the need, or to the matter of concern that has been noticed. At a collective level, just as establishing specific services marks a collective acceptance of responsibility for meeting the needs of, for example, young people experiencing mental health problems, developing and funding research programmes to seek better understanding and to come up with effective responses to such needs is an expression of collective responsibility. The preparedness of individuals and groups of researchers to work in this area also demonstrates a willingness to 'take care of' the causes of pain and injustice through applying research skills to contribute to a process of repair. As we negotiate the long-term consequences of the COVID-19 pandemic we all have cause to be grateful for researchers in many different disciplines taking responsibility for deepening knowledge and understanding of how best to respond, and to governments and other sources of funding committing resources to these projects.

But for those dependent on funding to make research happen the challenge is often to express their research plan in ways that both respects the matters of concern to those who are marginalised and to whom they have been attentive, and ways that are capable of 'fitting' funders' expectations. We both have much experience of failure in this respect. Sometimes it is clear that there is active resistance among powerful decision makers to attempts by researchers to address needs or identified problems through undertaking research that is framed in ways that can be challenging. In the 1990s Marian was a Mental Health Act Commissioner, visiting psychiatric hospitals where people were detained under the Mental Health Act. During that time she collaborated with a woman clinical psychologist working in a high-security hospital to develop a proposal that would have explored why the system was badly failing the women detained in these settings. This had also been the topic of an inquiry to which we had both given evidence. But it was clear that our aim of carrying out a detailed study with an explicitly feminist perspective was perceived as highly threatening, and, in spite of this being an area prioritised for research funding, we were blocked from proceeding. Service users seeking to develop their own research agendas and projects have faced particular difficulties in securing funding and then their work being discredited because of being carried out without recognised research funding (for example Staddon, 2012).

Doing research with care does not mean one person taking on or taking over responsibility for every aspect of the work. While holding overall responsibility for the effective conduct of work may lie with the person designated as Principal Investigator (PI), to interpret and act as if this means individual control over the process is as damaging as an individual carer 'sacrificing' themselves by taking over the life of a disabled person. Responsibility must focus on the different relationships involved as well as the technicalities of the research process. If research is to be a relational, caring process then all those involved in collaborative research teams have some responsibility for its conduct. This can generate dilemmas, particularly when power is unequally distributed among research partners. Sarah Banks and her colleagues write about those aspects of collaborative research that are rarely made visible when reports of projects are written up (Banks et al, 2019). One such example involved the need to remind a community group that receiving money to participate in a project meant this should be used for the research and not for other activities.

The ethical implications of caring relationships in which power is unequally distributed, but the contribution of all those involved is necessary to achieve the purpose to which care is directed, have received comparatively little attention. Nevertheless, this is an important aspect of the participative research practices we are advocating. It was recognised by those involved in community university research partnerships studied by Ceri Davies:

> Locating talk of emotions in relational ways of working was also demonstrated in a few examples in the context of 'care' for each other. Cara's interpretation of this was that she and her partners *have a shared responsibility to care for each other*. ... Lisa, a community partner at Island place also highlighted that people were working together because they were *interested in each other and they care about each other*. (Davies, 2016, p 178; original emphasis)

Responsibility also relates to the issue of accountability. Typically, researchers will be accountable to their funders and there will be mechanisms through which this is expressed: regular reporting and discussions with a steering group are common. But how do researchers give expression to their accountability to those they are researching or on whom they depend for the cooperation necessary to complete the work? And what about their responsibility for their colleagues and to their employers? These reflect the way in which research is seen as a collaborative effort – or not. But this is also impacted by the context in which the research is conducted and the extent to which the broader environment is one that understands the necessity of maintaining webs of care through the conduct of research.

Davies' (2016) study of research partnerships with different communities based in two universities in the UK and Canada was carried out in universities that had made public commitments to supporting research collaborations with local communities.[2] The specific initiatives Davies looked at were ones that were quite well established and proposed as examples of the type of partnerships the universities wished to support. Responsibility featured frequently in interviews as key to the conduct of such collaborations. It was linked to both trust and care:

> The dynamics of collaboration that respondents identified as being important included trust, reciprocity and mutual benefit. My data also

shows that some people talked about not just a commitment to the relationship but a responsibility for what people were doing and who they were doing it with. This was also accompanied by the presence of emotions and talked about in the context of 'care' for each other and the building of friendships. (Davies, 2016, p 173)

The significance of these relational values was reinforced by the focus of much of the research that Ceri was exploring, and the experiences of those involved in this. Evidence of the need for repair created a particular responsibility for ensuring the wellbeing of those involved. For example:

Abby, a community researcher in the Indigenous histories project at Island University talked about this in relation to how the group of young people she was working with were uncovering the stories of their relatives who had survived the residential school system: *'we did a lot of sharing circles too when we were all together we would just kind of like go around and talk about, just make sure everyone was ok. There was a lot of safety in that way, and support with each other'.* (Davies, 2016, p 175; original emphasis)

The residential school system referred to was one in which the children of indigenous people in Canada were removed from their communities to be educated according to culturally dominant values and methods. It contributed to a fracturing of communities, abuse, violence and a loss of indigenous culture. Davies invoked the concept of 'relational accountability' to characterise the way in which her informants involved in research partnerships with indigenous groups spoke of the type of relationships they considered necessary to sustain trusting and caring research partnerships. These could be threatened by actions on the part of others in the academic institutions that were seeking to promote and extend this way of working, but who did not always fully understand the implications of this.

Sarah goes on to highlight another aspect of how trust worked in relationships, and how crucial maintaining trust was. This was also about taking responsibility for ensuring the relational and trusting nature of the work was done with integrity. She identified a context in her institution where people are pushed to 'give up' their contacts to others in a department when they needed to evidence external relationships. Her issue with this approach was that different people approaching the same partners might not act or think in the same way as her and risk damaging the relationship. (Davies, 2016, p 174)

One way of seeking to ensure that responsibility is enshrined in working relationships is to establish a memorandum of understanding that addresses the ways in which different partners in the research will work together. But like all such formalised mechanisms, the implementation of such understandings requires the existence of trusting relationships and cannot on their own ensure shared responsibility.

Responsibility for the effective conduct of the work does not end with the completion of the research. There is also a responsibility for ensuring some positive impact. Promising that research has a potential to achieve beneficial change is often part of the process of gaining agreement to take part and failing to live up to that can not only damage those involved in the particular project, but undermine future trust in those seeking to undertake research in a similar area.

## Competence

Tronto's (2013) third phase of care, caregiving, is what is often thought of as 'what care is'. This is the hands-on work of care. It is associated with competence as a moral quality necessary for care. At its most fundamental it requires us to ask whether those who 'don't know what they're doing' should be undertaking whatever practice they are pursuing because an absence of competence means that the need for care cannot be met. In the context of research it prompts us to ask about the dangers of letting someone undertake a research project when they properly understand neither the methodological nor ethical issues at stake, or when they have insufficient understanding of the world into which they are entering to conduct themselves in a way that will not cause damage. Such competences go beyond knowing what is necessary to collect data and conduct analyses, either statistical or qualitative, that will generate valid results. In Haraway's PigeonBlog example (pp 56–57), the design of monitoring instruments needed to not only ensure accuracy of readings, but to be capable of being carried without risking harm to the birds.

As Ceri Davies' work demonstrated, a familiar competence in the conduct of research with people who are marginalised or oppressed concerns the process of negotiating access. Often this requires a personal knowledge and acceptability which then carries with it responsibilities to honour the trust that has been given. It is concern about this that caused Sarah (quoted in the previous section) to worry about being asked to share contact details to help other researchers access people she had worked with. Being competent means that you are able to demonstrate that competence at the right times when it is needed. But in partnerships where there are unknowns, competence also refers to knowing when to step back and be instructed about what to do, or what you do not know (Edwards et al, 2020). 'Professional' researchers may need to demonstrate humility and to recognise that they are dependent on the knowledge of others. This is counterintuitive in academic life where authority derives from expertise and knowledge. The ability to exercise attentive listening remains necessary throughout a project. So too does the capacity to 'deliberate with care' (Barnes, 2008) in contexts in which both what people have to say and the way in which they speak can challenge professional norms and assumptions. The deliberative process within collaborative research teams can be seen to reflect other forums in which people who are marginalised or oppressed seek to influence the process of policy making (Barnes, 2002; Ward and Barnes, 2015).

Competences can be developed through collaborative research practices that both recognise what people bring to the process, and build new competences through caring relationships within teams. Working with old people as co-researchers meant they developed competence in research itself, as well as bringing to the project not only experiential knowledge of growing older, but also competences from their younger lives and work as counsellors, social care managers, nurses and other occupations (Barnes et al, 2018). One of Marian's favourite experiences during this work was to observe a methodological challenge from one of our co-researchers to an academic presenter at a conference. The presenter looked surprised to be on the receiving end of a challenge from someone she did not expect to be competent in this area.

Just as responsibilities lie not only with the PI, careful, relational research requires us to think in terms of distributed and different competences and the ways in which these need to be woven together during the conduct of projects. Technical and relational competence can both develop through the process of working together. Reciprocal learning can develop in a context in which there is a preparedness both to show humility about limitations as well as share expertise.

The significance of the context in which research is undertaken has taken on a particular significance during the time in which we have been writing this book and has offered a particular challenge to ways in which we can research with care. Social distancing resulting from the COVID-19 pandemic has resulted in changes to how research is carried out. In many UK universities, all qualitative research was halted at the beginning of lockdown. Ethics committees required a move to online projects for any research that continued during this time. For many researchers, this feels as though a shift has occurred where there is no going back to pre-pandemic methods of face-to-face recruitment and data collection, or bringing people together physically for focus groups. Researchers have been sharing best practice about how to engage people well in online research internationally during disasters such as the pandemic through blogs or edited collections such as from Kara and Khoo (2020a, 2020b, 2020c).

There has been less critical examination as yet of the implications of moving qualitative research online, including who this excludes from research and how this changes the nature of research as a relational practice. One part of this is the opportunity to offer hospitality as a way of valuing and thanking people for their participation. It is one form of competence that is necessary for doing research with care. Hospitality is extremely important in many cultures, and in research serves to show appreciation and respect to those who participate. In the early days of the pandemic, Tula was concerned about continuing a research advisory group which brought together people in recent mental health crises. People who contribute to this group were continuing to face mental health challenges. Peer support is important within the group and meetings include a checking in with people that they are feeling OK to be there and take part. On occasion some people have just wanted to sit through the session when they feel unable to contribute directly. There was a level of care needed with the contributors that is impossible to gauge online.

Although the impact of the pandemic has speeded up the extent to which everyday activities are taking place online, not everyone is willing to forgo privacy for the conveniences of online technologies. Not everyone has access to or competence with the necessary technologies. In her discussion of the importance of corporeal presence for attentive listening, Sophie Bourgault highlighted the dangers of too great a reliance on distancing technologies developing in an education context:

> A good classroom discussion and civic debate must entail some sensorial involvement – and affective shared moment of attention paid to certain individuals, books or claims together, with all the unpredictability, vulnerability, discomfort and frustration that this can cause. Learning, for *both student and teacher*, is no mere transmission of information; it is a flesh and bone encountering of wonder, generosity, difference, boredom and conflict – in short it entails an immersion in all too human, social living. (2016, p 331; original emphasis)

The same applies to the diverse encounters that take place during research. The voices of some research participants will be silenced as a result of technological distancing. In our research, we are involved in many ways with older people who do not have the technology and who value face to face interactions over technology-facilitated discussions. While all but one of the conversations we draw on in Part II of this book took place via Zoom, this was not possible with one woman who had been a co-researcher on the older people and wellbeing project (Barnes et al, 2018). Now in her 90s she is blind and has difficulty in speaking following a stroke. An email exchange was a poor substitute for being able to meet face to face.

As we try to learn different ways of building trust and establishing relationships in a socially distanced context, we should not lose sight of the relational care required in research. What we suggest here is that all of the considerations we offer in this book are as relevant for online-based research activities as they are for more conventional means of data collection, and that the concerns we raise may need more attention in this new environment.

## Responsiveness

One of the important insights Tronto (1993) offered in her early work on care ethics was the necessity to include care receiving and the responsiveness of the recipient as necessary to the completion of care. This is the fourth phase of care. Once again we can consider this in terms of the different relationships that research brings into being. When we were researching with older people in order to understand how wellbeing is generated and sustained in old age, we (the university researchers) were committed to carrying out the work as a collaboration with older people who worked alongside us as researchers. We sought to enable our co-researchers to take on different roles that they felt able to do and felt comfortable with. In some cases that comprised virtually all aspects of the research process: planning, data collection, data analysis, dissemination. But not all felt able to do this. One woman did not want to undertake interviews, but offered her contribution in transcribing interview recordings, drawing on her experience as an audio typist. This was an important task, but one she undertook largely on her own. She rarely attended team meetings. When she decided she no longer felt able to continue in this role and withdrew from the project we were concerned that her separation from the rest of the team had meant she had been distressed by listening to what were sometimes quite sad stories because she was not part of the conversation the team had about them. Her response to what she heard did not become part of the collective conversation that enabled other team members to process what they were hearing and to feel part of a process capable of generating change. We were probably insufficiently attentive to her response to the content of interviews and its consequences to pre-empt her feeling that she no longer wanted to be involved.

There are now many accounts from service users about their experiences of being invited to be involved alongside academic researchers in carrying out research projects (for example Ostrer and Morris, 2009; Turner and Gillard, 2012). These responses to invitations to act as co-researchers may not be framed by reference to care ethics, but clearly demonstrate the importance of care in the conduct of research. While some find the experience of being involved in research 'empowering', for others it can be frustrating or worse. We also need to be aware of the impact for lone researchers of researching in areas they care about. The experiences of lone researchers and their capacity to care for themselves whist carrying out research are illustrated by Patsy Staddon's (2012) account of her research into women users of alcohol. Staddon was herself a recovered alcoholic and her research was intended to both explore women's experiences of alcohol services, and the views of service providers. She wrote of the high emotional risks she carried as she processed both the resonances in interviews to her own experiences, and her constant sense of having her own worth as a 'knower' questioned because of her history.

The response of researchers to the troubling things that they hear can impact both on those who share these experiences and those who do not. Because researchers may care about the issues they research they can be touched by what they learn from this process. While the precise dynamics may be different depending on the existence or not of shared experiences, this is not an argument for excluding those with experience, or not, from carrying out particular projects. Faulkner and Tallis (2009, p 54) argue that shared experience both of the experience of mental illness and of being the object of research, can enhance the care taken in designing projects to minimise harms: 'The findings demonstrate the considerable care and concern shown by service user and survivor researchers in undertaking research. Many based their current practice on their own experience of "being researched" and treated as research fodder without the respect of others that they would now advocate.'

Ceri Davies (2016, p 179) wrote of researchers with indigenous people in Canada recognising the importance of listening to those recounting bad experiences of research. She cites Wilson and Wilson (1998), 'who argue that a researcher should fulfil his or her relationship with the world around him or her, by making careful choices about their work that can be accountable to people, traditions, the earth and spirit'. She also highlights the indigenous concept of 'a good way' which was cited to denote participation that honours tradition and spirit. Here Davies is quoting a researcher working with indigenous people living with HIV/AIDS:

> That relational accountability and ... knowing that communities can come back to us and say 'that wasn't done in a good way' or 'I have an issue with the way this was done'. ... And I think for communities to be able to say to us that they feel comfortable with us. ... I mean that is our purpose right – to hear their voice, to have their input, to have their – what they're saying. (2016, p 176)

This approach included being mindful that people were recognised and supported to say how they felt about their experiences and for this to carry weight in how the collaboration happened.

One outcome of the project that Faulkner and Tallis (2009) cite was the development of guidelines for ethical survivor research. The first principle of this was that '[s]urvivor research should attempt to counter the stigma and discrimination experienced by survivors in society' (p 55). This is an explicit statement of the necessity for research and researchers to be focused on 'repair' as they carry out research. Our argument in this book is that this applies equally to research carried out by others as well as by those with lived experience. This is not solely a matter of possible self-interest: those of us who have not so far experienced mental distress cannot guarantee that we will never do so; most of us do hope to live into old age so want to experience old age as a good time. The care ethics principle of solidarity, of caring with others, is one that not only argues for an openness to experiences that we do not share, but is essential for the development of the collective responsibility that underpins caring democracies (Tronto, 2013).

## Solidarity

Thus, we come to Tronto's (2013) final phase of care. Research that is designed and carried out in a way that builds awareness and sensitivity to others' responses both to the issues being researched and to the processes involved in increasing knowledge and understanding of these issues, is not complete without considering how it can build solidarity. In the first instance this means solidarity among those directly involved in the research itself: the research team, those who are the focus of research and those who commission it. This is one of the key benefits of working with others different from ourselves in carrying out the work. The process of designing a project, collecting data, trying to make sense of it and then working out how to communicate what we have learnt to those who need to know, contains the possibility of increasing our understanding of the circumstances of others; of giving recognition to others whose life experiences and competences offer different ways of thinking about and being in the world; of recognising different kinds of knowledge that have been suppressed or devalued; and of enabling self-reflection as a result of our encounters with those differences.

This is important not only to understand what is needed as people work together in carrying out research, but also when we think about the contribution of research to broader social change. What do we do with the understanding and knowledge that we generate through research? And it is here that we move directly into the contested and thorny question of 'impact'. As we expand the practical implications of the phases of care to the doing of research we demonstrate the integrity of care that Tronto wrote of in *Moral Boundaries*. Her later addition of a fifth phase of care, 'caring with', perhaps embodies what we mean by the type of research we are emphasising here. 'Researching with' rather than 'on' people directs our attention to the necessity of ethical practice that goes well beyond effective completion of ever more complex forms necessary to receive ethical approval for a specific research project, and takes this into our responsibilities to others to make a difference as a result of the work we have done and the input we have asked of them. The principle linked to caring with/researching with is that of solidarity. This solidarity is not one born out of pity for others and contains, as Hoggett (2006) has argued, often contradictory views about the particular individuals with whom we may have been working. But it derives from a commitment, a caring about, that links this to an awareness of injustice and a drive towards action capable of repair.

Common to early developments in participatory or emancipatory research in all contexts was not only that research should connect with lived experience, but that it should be a purposive activity with beneficial change as its aim. One observation of researchers who have been using participatory approaches for some time, is that the excitement associated with earlier actions that promised transformative outcomes has fizzled out. People who have experience of the issue being researched see no actual impact and become disillusioned with research as a means for change. They see large research grants resulting in little action – writing research papers just does not cut it, and reflect that the research money could have been better used to improve the quality of the lives of those affected more directly. This is a harsh reality for those of us committed to research, but it is a response that needs to be addressed. Large funding bodies in some areas (such as health research in the UK) require researchers to involve people with experiential knowledge in both creating research proposals and in governance processes throughout research projects. Funders recognise the need for research projects to impact on practice, and impact plans are expected that inform how this may happen. Some funders offer additional funds for this, including activities that improve broader engagement through the use of media or artist involvement to communicate the project to a non-academic audience. One example of this was the commissioning of art work intended to communicate what it is like to be an old person having to negotiate the system of self-funding for social care, based on research carried out in Brighton, Solihull and Lincoln.[3] The challenges of ensuring that participatory research can and does generate valuable legacies was a particular focus for work conducted in the 'Connected Communities' programme in the UK (Facer and Pahl, 2017). Their adoption of the term 'legacy' rather than 'impact' was intended to reflect both the problematic way in which linear models of impact failed to encompass the messy and diffuse ways in which research can make a difference, but also the importance of recognising that collaborative inquiry cannot be complete without attending to 'what is left behind' (Facer and Pahl, 2017, p 226).

From an ethics of care perspective we need to think impact, or legacy, and solidarity together. We need to bring a time perspective into this – thinking of the immediate relational impacts that research can and does have on those who are directly involved; the much longer timescales during which we might need patience in understanding what is required to achieve good change – and when we need to be impatient about failures to act and respond. In order to think about these issues we return to Carol Gilligan, to Donna Haraway and Maria Puig de la Bellacasa as well as to the experiences of those we have worked with and the topics we have worked on.

In her book *Joining the Resistance*, Carol Gilligan (2011) 'looks back to look forward'. She revisits the factors that led her to write *In a Different Voice* and recounts her journey from psychology to politics as she develops her argument about the enduring and increasing importance of care ethics. Writing this during the COVID-19 lockdown, her words are prophetic:

> In an age of climate change, pandemics, and nuclear weapons, interdependence has become self-evident. And with this recognition it becomes obvious as Patricia Papperman writes, that 'There is nothing exceptional about vulnerable people.' Vulnerability, once associated with women, is a characteristic of humans.
>
> Looking forward then, we can expect a struggle. … Once the ethic of care is released from its subsidiary position within a justice framework, it can guide us by framing the struggle in a way that clarifies what is at stake and by illuminating a path of resistance grounded not in ideology but in our humanity. (Gilligan, 2011, pp 42–43)

The public discourse of 2020/2021 is replete with references to interdependence, care and vulnerability. Pundits from left and right opine that the world will be transformed by the shared experience of the impact of an invisible enemy that respects neither gender nor nationality – though has more ravaging effects on those already made vulnerable by illness. But we know already that immediate and real experiences of the virus and its consequences are hugely unequal and that the longer-term consequences are exposing and exacerbating many dimensions of inequality and vulnerability, including those of race, poverty and occupation. Positive transformations will only come from including those most impacted in decisions about how to move forward.

The work of 'illuminating a path of resistance' is a continuing one that requires collaboration, attention and action. Gilligan's reflections on how she got to hear the different voice through which ethical dilemmas are expressed are important. They remind us that how we know involves the humility of acknowledging what we don't know at any point in time, as well as how we might rework and renew our understandings through the things we learn with and from others. We have tried to do some of that work in this book by reflecting on aspects of our own research that might, as Sevenhuijsen (2003) suggests in relation to policy analysis, be subject to 'renewal' from an ethic of care. We suggest that this process is best done in conversation with others. And we have been suggesting throughout this book that those others include both researchers from different disciplines who can encourage us to go beyond our own ways of looking at the world, and those who do not think of themselves as researchers but help us engage in what Puig de la Bellacasa (2017) calls the 'disruptive thought of care' (p 1).

Those conversations have an impact – they are transformative in their own right and they can build solidarity between people who may not otherwise have come into contact with each other. Ceri Davies again:

> The examples from my data where collaborations contained a '*huge relational component ...*' brought with it relationships that extended to '*becoming part of each other's lives*' (Cara). There were examples across both fieldwork sites where people's relationships extended to developing friendships with some of their partners. Lisa at Island place for example reflected on this in our interview: '*... the relationship extends beyond a professional relationship and all of a sudden you become friends*'. (2016, p 178; original emphasis)

From our own work we can offer examples of people from mental health user groups, from carers' organisations, older people with whom we collaborated on research projects who not only contributed to our thinking at the time of the initial project, but with whom we developed ongoing professional and personal relationships and who have continued to be a point of reference – both in person and as we reflect on what worked well and what troubled us in our research, as we have thought about our work but also how we have tried to live our lives. In Marian's case, more recent work with a woman with a strong Christian faith in researching what a faith-based community has meant to those who have been part of it did not lead to a 'conversion', but did offer both a renewed respect for those for whom faith is the basis of care and recognition of what this can contribute to recovery for many experiencing the impacts of addictions and mental illness (Barnes et al, 2022). These personal solidarities spread out. We take them into other conversations, use them in spaces in which we seek to make a difference. And we recognise the way they impact on how we try to research in future.

The vast range of disciplinary and topic focused work that starts from or employs care ethics in some way encourages us to explore inter or post disciplinary solidarities in our research. So let us look beyond our (Tula's and Marian's) areas of expertise to consider how others work with care in ways that can help us build the impact of our research in the context of interdependence and shared vulnerabilities.

We have noted that the arts and humanities are one sphere within which solidaristic research relationships can and are being expanded and in Part II we develop discussion of projects involving the use of creative methods in both conducting and disseminating research. The telling of stories using a variety of media – poetry, photography, theatre or other means – can engage attention and prompt responses to lives very different to our own. But drawing on the work of Puig de la Bellacasa (2017), we want to suggest the potential for careful research that promotes solidarities beyond those between and among *people*, and that encompasses things that are interconnected in a web of care, but which too rarely receive attention. Our starting point in this book is the necessity of caring about and including in research those who are marginalised, oppressed or subject to a range of injustices. Puig de la Bellacasa (2017, p 170) writes: 'It is partly because of the devalued significance of care that feminist research on practices of care is often oriented by an ethico-political commitment to investigate the significance of neglected things, practises and experiences made invisible or marginalised by dominant 'successful', (technoscientific) mobilizations'. Being attentive to neglected things can enable their significance to be demonstrated and their role in care to be made visible. Brian Davey's spoof email about Ecoworks contained more than a grain of truth about the significance of the allotment to the empowerment of mental health service users. For Puig de la Bellacasa the neglected thing that her words introduce is soil:

> Attention to ways in which notions of 'soil care' could potentially be transformed in these times of environmental unsettledness brings to light possible alternative practical, ethical and affective ecologies. I therefore engage with soil as matters of care: human–soil relations of care and soil ontologies are entangled. What soil is thought to be affects the way in which it is cared for, and vice versa, modes of care have effects in what soil becomes. (Puig de la Bellacasa, 2017, p 170)

To research soil and to demonstrate the impact of the way in which soil is thought of by humans, and cared for, or not, as a result, requires engaging with soil science, well beyond what we understand as social science. But this, in turn, connects with the economics of agricultural production, the cultural study of rural life and the literal and metaphorical evocation of soil in art and literature. Had I and my colleagues been sufficiently attentive to the significance of Ecoworks we might have found ourselves needing to understand the way in which the soil bacterium *mycobacterium vaccae* activates the same serotonin-releasing neurons in the brain as are targeted by the drug Prozac (Lewis-Stempel, 2016, p 86).

The significance of the enrichment of soil and its connection both to natural cycles of growth and decay, and to the work required in recovery from addiction or mental illness, was captured by a former warden of a residential community that supports those seeking such recovery:

> And to engage with the land as well and the rhythms of life and death and new life emerging and how that reflected some of the things that

were happening for people in terms of what did they have to let go of or die to and where might new life emerge for them, and we often made quite a bit of manure really, because it's a great metaphor that, how manure can be a source of life and how we work with the crap of people's lives and how that can somehow generate new life really. (Barnes et al, 2022, p 187)

And from the same study another former community member spoke of the web of care encompassing people, crop growing and food production:

I did a lot of cooking ... every meal it was a way of caring for people in a practical way, in a physical way. ... I loved going in the garden and getting stuff, when it appeared I loved thinking, well, Henry grew the beans. ... I loved the way everybody's place in the making of the meal, it's not the person who cooks but everybody who had a role in it appearing. ... I wanted people to be healthy and whole, but sometimes they'd been so neglected and neglectful of themselves that actually that kind of caring is a very uplifting thing. (Barnes, 2019a, p 146)

This study of the Pilsdon Community draws together an awareness of the interconnectedness of people and things within their environment that both contribute to care, but also need to be cared for (Barnes, 2019a). Research that attends to such connections helps us think of ourselves as interdependent not only with other people, but also with other species, with the land and with plants. Thinking about such connections with care is the opposite of thinking about how we can exploit these resources to sustain ourselves, but what we need to do to sustain these connections. It drives us towards solidarity rather than exploitation.

## Conclusion

In these first four chapters we have built an argument for approaching research as a caring practice. We have emphasised the importance of recognising the contribution of different people involved in different ways to building knowledge and understanding through research, and we have highlighted some of the ways in which that has been a source of troubles to those who have tried to develop more collaborative research practices. Even when researchers are motivated by care for the injustices experienced by others it can be hard to work together in ways that enable all to feel cared for. Care is a practice as well as an ethical way of thinking about interdependency and its political implications. Work on the ethics of care has emphasised the importance of being attentive to specific contexts and of working out how to do care that 'fits' the relational circumstances in which we live and work. This is best illustrated by example. So we have drawn from our own and others' experiences as we have built our argument. In the next part of the book we explore in more detail how others have tried to work with care ethics in carrying out their research.

# PART II

## Introduction to Part II: research as praxis

In Part I, we introduced the elements and phases of care and how these can be applied to research practice. These elements and phases, in our view, are always underpinned by the feminist concerns of justice and equality and are enacted in an attempt to achieve this. In research, as in other contexts, care is purposive. But justice and equality for whom, and how might those involved in research understand this? In this part of the book we explore and expand care ethics thinking and its application to research carried out with and by different groups of people whose experiences can help us better understand its significance. We do this by drawing on conversations with a diverse group of people who all have experience of care ethics in research. Whereas in Chapter 4 we structured our discussion by reference to phases of care, in this part we use the stages of research to reflect more deeply on the issues we are discussing.

An initial research idea can be a lightbulb moment or a slow-burn realisation. In the former, the switch is flicked and the issue comes into view – we recognise its importance. We also see what we do not know, what remains in the shadows and what we need to better understand. As we extend our knowledge of previous research and build our connections with those affected by the topic, the initial idea takes a firmer shape until we have a proposal we can use to secure the relevant support to get a project off the ground. In this part of the book we explore more about how these decisions are reached, who is included in generating ideas, and how these evolve and respond to different influences and perspectives. Do researchers draw on their own experiences, how do they work with people in more and less formal ways at the ideas stage and as the research develops? We ask how researchers are attentive to the people who contribute to research and how attentiveness can improve the experiences of involvement for people and the quality of the research itself.

The research we discuss here has been undertaken in different types of research partnerships or collaborations. Projects have adopted different methods to knowledge construction, including creative approaches to enable a flattening of hierarchies and avoid reliance on written or textual approaches. They include our own work where we have adopted ethics of care as a systematic guide and revision of research practices, as well as the work of others. As we discussed in Chapter 3 there are many different individuals and groups who have a connection with a research project: not only the researchers themselves and those they invite to take part, but also ethics committees, university research departments, budget holders, website controllers, publishers and academic journal editors, funders, media and other academic colleagues. What accountability, what attentiveness do we owe to these different groups? How do we negotiate our different responsibilities as researchers? If we care about a topic and want to make a difference what impact does this have on the way we navigate our responsibilities to, for example, co-researchers and funders? How many forms of responsibility can cohabit in this way and how do we acknowledge them? People are acutely aware of what they care about and whether the actions undertaken by researchers demonstrate a similar concern. Do we accept responsibility to contribute to repairing previous damage, to establish a new path for people that signifies a change from the past?

It is perhaps easy to accept the necessity for competence in carrying out research. But what forms of competence are needed to work in different contexts and how might they be distributed and developed among those taking part? In partnerships between researchers in the global north and global south, how do the principles of decoloniality influence the way we research together? People may not want to contribute to research projects, but their voices would significantly contribute to knowledge. So we look at the ways in which research may encourage and deter people whose voice is necessary.

Then how do we think about the way we encourage responsiveness from research participants? Some voices may not be easy to accept. They may be angry, people may not have verbal skills, or prefer to tell stories rather than answer questions. The structures we work in may offer up roles that do not make sense to those we invite to work with us. We invite them because of what we know about them, but they may want to take part because of an experience about which we know nothing. Can we make space to enable an expansive coming together and development of competence, contribution and perspective? We consider how the ethics of care's focus on responsiveness surfaces a responsibility to ensure that we are all open to change as we listen and hear from others.

And how might research generate solidarity? A focus on solidarity and trust returns us to the question of the axes along which this develops through the practices of research. The feminist origins of the care ethics encourage us to listen to different voices, especially those that have been silenced or unheard, to understand the consequences of harms that have been experienced, and to play our part in repairing those harms. But what does this mean in terms of the relationships we need to forge with others who are powerful, with our funders or employers, with those we need to influence to achieve change? How may the way we navigate these tensions and conflicts be guided through care ethics thinking?

There are a lot of questions here! We need many experiences to help us work out some ways through the dilemmas we face. We asked people involved in research who we knew had explicitly drawn on care ethics in their work, and/or who had committed to participative research, to contribute to discussions about researching with care to include their ideas and experiences in the following chapters. Although researchers may be influenced by care ethics, this may not always be explicit in the way they describe the methodologies they use. We wanted to invite people to address this directly and offer reflections that they might not have written about in books and articles. We wanted to understand how care ethics can be applied in topics and contexts different from those with which we are familiar and whether this way of thinking could help people improve their practice.

In the next three chapters we work through the doing of research in light of how we and others have used the ethics of care to inform and guide practices. We evolve the conceptualisations of Tronto's phases of care (1993, 2013) as applied to the making of new knowledge, with a view to extending our understanding of what careful research practice looks like. When we spoke with her, Umut Erel suggested that there is no existing book that informs thinking about careful research in practice. Here we begin to examine in more detail what these practices involve and what we and other researchers have learnt about them.

During our conversations people made links between personal stories and research topics. They spoke of motivations for researching that would make a difference. They sought to engage others in the research in ways that recognised potential vulnerabilities. They considered care and relationality – how the research could be developed in a way that cares for the people involved and enables people to contribute as they wish and are able to; what is necessary to welcome and appreciate the contributions people have to offer. Paying attention to the details of people's lives, the effort involved to participate, and the reasons why people want to be there, creates an atmosphere of care.

We draw on conversations with the following people:

*Bunty Bateman* worked with Marian, Bea Gahagan and Lizzie Ward on a project on older people and wellbeing in Brighton and Hove, UK. At the time she became involved Bunty was a volunteer for the local Age UK. She had a long history of voluntary work and community activism and had also been a union activist. She played a full part in the research, being a regular attender at research group meetings, undertaking interviews and focus groups, analysing transcripts and presenting findings at a range of events following the completion of the research. She spoke at the time about the tension she felt in her different roles as research interviewer and counsellor/advocate for older people. She also took part in a Knowledge Exchange project that generated filmed learning resources from the project, and she was involved in preparing a publication based on research findings by older people for older people, called 'As Time Goes By'. Her experience on this project led to her involvement in a range of other research projects and in training for health and social care workers. Sadly, Bunty died a few months after the conversation for this book. She was 90. At her funeral it was noted that she had been transcribing research interviews the day before she died.

*Vivienne Bozalek* has made a significant contribution to work on the ethics of care and has explored in depth the concept of privileged irresponsibility. We first met her when we organised a conference at the University of Brighton in 2012 where she gave a paper. She subsequently contributed a chapter on privilege and responsibility in a South African context to our edited book (Bozalek, 2015). Viv studied for her PhD with Selma Sevenhuijsen and initially taught and researched in relation to social work. In this context she developed both a critical perspective on social work and its relationship to social justice, and a particular interest in pedagogy. Her more recent work has been more directly focused on the latter. As well as these areas of interest we wanted to talk with her about her recent work drawing from feminist new materialism and post-humanism. Viv's current work is about post-qualitative research methodologies, drawing on the work of Donna Haraway and Karen Barad as inspiration for how research may be conducted differently. This is about how research practices can render each person capable, enhancing participation and research data. Viv's work is different from that of others we spoke with in its engagement with some quite difficult theoretical material that emphasises the importance of 'thinking with' care, rather than the 'doing with' participatory research practices that have been the focus for most of this book (for example Bozalek and Zembylas, 2017). Now a Professor Emerita, Viv continues to write and inspire both colleagues and students – as well as swimming with octopuses near her home in South Africa.

*Ceri Davies* was working for the National Centre for Social Research when we spoke to her. Her job as Director of the Centre for Deliberative Research involves her in leading teams of researchers as well as coordinating what are sometimes large-scale and complex deliberative projects exploring a range of policy issues. Previously she had worked at the University of Brighton for Community-University Partnership Programme (CUPP) where she had a key role in facilitating research partnerships between academics and community groups. Ceri had initially been interested in natural sciences, but a research project in Uganda turned her attention to how communities are involved in decisions regarding their communities. This fitted well with her community and local action. While at Brighton she undertook a PhD, supervised by Marian, that examined case studies of collaborative research between universities in England and Canada. Her thesis was titled: 'Whose

Knowledge Counts? Exploring Cognitive Justice in Community-University Collaborations'. The projects she looked at in Canada involved collaborations with indigenous peoples and offered particularly important insights into many of the issues we are exploring in this book – we have already cited some of her findings in previous chapters. A key dilemma for her as a doctoral student was the feasibility of using participatory methods, particularly in the context of fieldwork that had to be conducted in a limited period of time in another country.

*Umut Erel* worked at the Open University and held a Chair in Sociology. Her research employs an intersectional approach and explores how gender, migration and ethnicity inform practices of citizenship. She first developed this work in her PhD where she looked at skilled migrant women from Turkey in Britain and Germany. Umut herself had migrated with her family from Turkey to Germany where she lived before moving to the UK. She explored migrant experiences further in the context of paid and unpaid work of refugee women in the voluntary sector and migrants in new areas of multiculture. She has drawn on care ethics in considering the relationship between care and citizenship and has adopted participatory research methods in her work. Her research projects include: 'Participatory Arts and Social Action Research: Participatory Theatre and Walking Methods', with Maggie O'Neill and Tracey Reynolds. She received an Arts and Humanities Research Council Networking Grant for a project called 'Migrant Mothers Caring for the Future: Creative Interventions into Citizenship', also carried out with Tracey Reynolds, and 'Migration Making People, Making Places' with Jacqueline Broadhead and Giles Mohan. Umut talked about experiences of working on these projects in her conversation with us, reflecting both on the significance of her personal background in motivating interest and the professional challenges associated with working in genuinely participatory ways in the context of other pressures in academic life.

*Ruth Evans* has a long-standing interest in the lives of children and young people who care for disabled parents, older relatives and other family members, both in the UK and in sub-Saharan Africa (for example Evans, 2012). She also contributed to the 'Critical Care' conference in Brighton and to the subsequent book (Evans, 2015). She is a human geographer, with a background in gender, development and social studies of childhood currently holding a Chair at the University of Reading. Ruth developed participatory methods in her doctoral research in Tanzania and subsequently worked as a research fellow on the National Evaluation of the Children's Fund (see Chapter 3) and was involved in the development of participatory methods in that context, as well as further developing video and other participatory art methods in her own work. Ruth's research has used the ethics of care as a way of understanding young caregiving and relationality within families, the construction of good care practices and the support that families are able to access through the state and other agencies. Ruth has been highlighting how young people and children are active participants in practices of care, often in difficult circumstances, challenging the prevalent view of adult–child caregiving and perceptions of 'family troubles'. The ethics of care has been helpful in analysing the gendered and generational dynamics of everyday familial caring responsibilities in diverse contexts and the devaluing of care work. Her recent work, that she spoke about during our conversation, has focused on experiences of bereavement, inheritance and care in Senegal, Ghana, Uganda and Tanzania and care and support among refugees and other migrants in the UK. She led a Leverhulme Trust research project on bereavement, care and family relations in urban Senegal which explicitly adopted an ethic of care approach to the topic and methodology. This work raises a number of practical and ethical challenges associated with north–south research collaborations, as well as those associated with the translation of concepts and questions of cultural understanding. In her conversation Ruth reflected on these professional issues associated with the practice of careful, respectful research and interpreting family struggles across north–south boundaries, as well as some of the more personal factors impacting the research we do. During her academic career Ruth has developed a different understanding about her own life and how this related to her field of research. She calls for more care for research teams and advocates supervision and debriefing for researchers working with difficult topics. As Ruth's reflections indicate, we may not always be fully aware of the connections between the 'personal' and 'professional' when we start out, but we may become more aware through the work we do.

*Beatrice Gahagan* met and worked with Marian when they both 'inherited' a joint university/Age UK project on older people and alcohol. A collaborative relationship between the University of Brighton and the local Age UK had existed for some time. Bea, who holds a doctorate in psychology, was then a senior manager with Age UK with responsibilities that included both service management and development. They continued to work together on the alcohol project and then, with Lizzie Ward, jointly developed the proposal for the older people and wellbeing project. The context for this was an unusual one. The Chief Officer of Age UK at the time approached the university with an offer of funding for research if the university agreed to match it. It would be up to the relevant university staff to determine the topic in collaboration with Bea. The wellbeing project was thus developed 'from the ground up' with a degree of flexibility not often available when needing to bid for research funds. Bea had a key role in recruiting and supporting older people as co-researchers in this project, as well as contributing to the planning and conduct of the research, and liaising with local practitioners. Changes in personnel within Age UK led eventually to Bea leaving her post. She continued to work with Lizzie Ward on another research project and is now working in training and staff development roles within Brighton and Hove City Council. She reflected on the strength she felt she gained from working with the ethics of care and the ways in which this had helped her confidence in the robustness of the values she seeks to uphold in her work.

It was not possible to talk directly to *Liz Ray*, who was also a co-researcher on the older people and wellbeing project. Liz is now blind and lives in a residential home where a member of staff facilitated an email exchange about her involvement in this project with her. Like Bunty, Liz played a full part in the research. Among her previous roles she had been a magistrate and a volunteer for Age UK.

And some more about us:

*Tula*: my research started at the University of Birmingham when I was a mental health nurse working in practice with people with mental health conditions and dementia. As a mental health nurse, I was critical of service provision in its failure to meet the needs of people. When I read Joan Tronto's and Selma Sevenhuijsen's work during my PhD study, my initial reaction was how valuable that thinking was to guide and review practice. Ethics of care has since been a way of thinking about the world that enables a different engagement and consideration of everyday practices. My initial research examined the practices of nurses and social workers and how people with dementia were included in decisions that were made about moving into residential care. This used an ethics of care as an analytical framework. I researched disability and mental health issues alongside people with experience through SureSearch at the University of Birmingham. When I moved to Aotearoa New Zealand in 2006 I worked with people with experience and in partnership with Māori in research and education. Research projects included community-based alcohol and other drug service delivery for young people aged 12–16 at risk of out of home placement; acceptability of residential care life to people with dementia; and mental health activists' priorities for change. Back in the UK from 2015 to 2021, research included a participatory project about the acceptability of Global Positioning System (GPS) tracking devices for people with dementia with Ruth Bartlett; partnership work between indigenous and non-indigenous researchers and communities; and the co-production of a self- management app with people using mental health crisis services. More recently, I have been considering the democratisation of research and what the ethics of care can contribute to careful research. I am a steering group member on the international Care Ethics Research Consortium, and a member of the Multispecies Dementia Network. In 2021, as we were writing this book, I returned to Aotearoa New Zealand. All my research has been guided by the ethics of care, especially when I have encountered challenges in the doing of the research. A good example would be a partnership with Māori to guide responses that aim to avoid any echoes of coloniality when working with indigenous people.

*Marian*: I am now retired and have a long period as a researcher to look back on. As Tula and I have talked about this book I have reflected on aspects of that work I recognise as significant personally, politically and professionally. The significance of some things has become more apparent as I have grown older and have more direct experience of care in diverse contexts. I have also learnt from others' work on feminist care ethics that has inspired and stimulated me, and from people doing care in often very difficult circumstances. I have researched a wide range of topics during my life and have done so in different contexts: as an employee of local authority social services departments; as a researcher on others' projects and as PI; in large and small teams; carrying out small pieces of solo unfunded work, and, most recently, as a volunteer involved in an oral history of a residential community. There are two projects that I want to say a bit about here: in a way they can be regarded as 'bookends' to my research career.

I worked on an evaluation of the Birmingham Community Care Special Action Project in the early 1990s. This was an early example of an initiative to develop inter-agency and user-led services. It involved a series of projects working with disabled people, mental health service users and unpaid carers. It seemed obvious to me that the evaluation should also adopt participative methods and the most extended aspect of that was work with two groups of carers. I invited carers who had taken part in consultations to work with me to develop criteria for assessing action following consultation, and in establishing ways of monitoring progress. I went into this without any pre-defined ways of working, nor with any insights from practical and theoretical work on participative research methods. At the start I said to carers that I did not know precisely how it would go, but asked if they were up for trying this with me. A key thing I learnt was the necessity of making space for people to talk with each other about things happening in their lives – this could not be a solely task-focused process. From that I learnt the importance of the relational dimension of research and how this can build solidarity.

A final project during my working life is the project on wellbeing that Bea, Bunty and Liz were involved in and about which we say quite a bit during this book. This was an opportunity to put into practice a range of learning from previous work, an opportunity greatly enhanced by working with great collaborators and in a context that enabled considerable flexibility. It was also an opportunity to work both with insights into participative research, and from care ethics. I was hooked from the start by Selma Sevenhuijsen's 1998 book, *Citizenship and the Ethics of Care: Feminist Considerations on Justice, Morality and Politics*. The introductory chapter to this starts with an observation of a care worker 'schmoozing' an elderly woman. It is rare to find a discussion of ethical and political theory that starts with everyday life in a care home. It seems to me appropriate that one of my final pieces of research enabled me to bring home my commitments to participatory research by also addressing the experience of growing old from an ethics of care perspective.

We would like to thank Bea, Bunty, Ceri, Ruth, Umut and Viv for their generosity in time and expertise joining us in discussions about care and research. We have included examples from these discussions in each of the chapters to illuminate how care ethics thinking can change perspectives on research and provide guidance for working out situations that challenge us which may present from all the different interested parties in research. We have also included references for further reading from these and other care ethicists that we think will support theoretical development of ethics of care in research.

## Selected reading on care from us and the people we spoke to

Barnes, M. (2006) *Caring and Social Justice*, Basingstoke: Palgrave.

Barnes, M. (2011) 'Abandoning care? A critical perspective on personalisation from an ethic of care', *Ethics and Social Welfare*, 5(2), 153–167.

Barnes, M. (2018) 'Getting out of line: Reflections on ageing activism and moral agency', *Ethics and Social Welfare*, 12(3), 204–215.

Barnes, M. (2019a) 'Community care: The ethics of care in a residential community', *Ethics and Social Welfare*, 14(2), 140–155.

Barnes, M. (2019b) 'Old age and caring democracy' in H. Tam (ed) *Whose Government Is It? The Renewal of State-Citizen Cooperation*, Bristol: Policy Press, pp 143–158.

Barnes, M. and Brannelly, T. (2008) 'Achieving care and social justice for people with dementia', *Nursing Ethics*, 15(3), 384–395.

Barnes, M. and Henwood, F. (2015) 'Inform with care: Ethics and information in care for people with dementia', *Ethics and Social Welfare*, 9(2), 147–163.

Barnes, M., Brannelly, T., Ward, L. and Ward, N. (2015) *Ethics of Care: Critical Advances in International Perspectives*, Bristol: Policy Press.

Barnes, M., Gahagan, B. and Ward, L. (2018) *Re-imagining Old Age: Wellbeing, Care and Participation*, Wilmington, DE: Vernon Press.

Barnes, M., Davies, M. and Prior, D. (2022) *Living Life in Common: Stories from the Pilsdon Community*, Leicester: Matador.

Bozalek, V. and Zembylas, M. (2017) 'Diffraction or reflection? Sketching the contours of two methodologies in educational research', *International Journal of Qualitative Studies in Education*, 30(2), 111–127.

Bozalek, V., Bayat, A., Motala, S., Mitchell, V. and Gachago, D. (2016) 'Diffracting socially just pedagogies through stained glass', *South African Journal of Higher Education*, 30(3), 201–218.

Bozalek, V., Zembylas, M., Motala, S. and Holscher, D. (eds) (2021) *Higher Education Hauntologies: Living with Ghosts for a Justice-to-Come*, London: Routledge.

Brannelly, T. (2011) 'That others matter: The moral achievement – care ethics and citizenship in practice with people with dementia', *Ethics and Social Welfare*, 5(2), 210–216.

Brannelly, T. (2016) 'Citizenship and people living with dementia: A case for the ethics of care', *Dementia*, 15(3), 304–314.

Brannelly, T. (2018) 'An ethics of care research manifesto', *International Journal of Care and Caring*, 2(3), 367–378.

Brannelly, T. and Boulton, A. (2017) 'The ethics of care and transformational research practices in Aotearoa New Zealand', *Qualitative Research*, 17(3), 340–350.

Brannelly, T., Boulton, A. and Te Hiini, A. (2013) 'A relationship between the ethics of care and Māori worldview: The place of relationality and care in Maori mental health service provision', *Ethics and Social Welfare*, 7(4), 410–422.

Edwards, R. and Brannelly, T. (2017) 'Approaches to democratising qualitative research methods', *Qualitative Research*, 17(3), 271–277.

Edwards, R., Barnes, H., McGregor, D. and Brannelly, T. (2020) 'Supporting Indigenous and non-Indigenous research partnerships', *The Qualitative Report*, 25(13), 6–15.

Erel, U. (2013) '"Troubling" or "ordinary"? Children's views on migration and intergenerational ethnic identities' in J. Ribbens McCarthy, C. Hooper and V. Gillies (eds) *Family Troubles? Exploring Changes and Challenges in the Family Lives of Children and Young People*, Bristol: Policy Press, pp 199–208.

Erel, U. (2018) 'Saving and reproducing the nation: Struggles around right-wing politics of social reproduction, gender and race in austerity Europe', *Women's Studies International Forum*, 68, 173–182.

Erel, U., Reynolds, T. and Kaptani, E. (2017) 'Participatory theatre for transformative social research', *Qualitative Research*, 17(3), 302–312.

Erel, U., Reynolds, T. and Kaptani, E. (2018) 'Migrant mothers creative interventions into racialised citizenships', *Ethnic and Racial Studies*, 41(1), 55–72.

Evans, R. (2011a) '"We are managing our own lives ...": Life transitions and care in sibling-headed households affected by AIDS in Tanzania and Uganda', *Area*, 43(4), 384–396.

Evans, R. (2011b) 'Young caregiving and HIV in the UK: Caring relationships and mobilities in African migrant families', *Population, Space and Place*, 17(4), 338–360.

Evans, R. (2012) 'Sibling caringscapes: Time-space practices of caring within youth-headed households in Tanzania and Uganda', *Geoforum*, 43(4), 824–835.

Evans, R. (2014) 'Parental death as a vital conjuncture? Intergenerational care and responsibility following bereavement in Senegal', *Social & Cultural Geography*, 15(5), 547–570.

Evans, R. (2015) 'Negotiating intergenerational relations and care in diverse African contexts' in R. Vanderbeck and N. Worth (eds) *Intergenerational Space*, London: Routledge, pp 199–213.

Evans, R. (2017) 'Caring after parental death: Sibling practices and continuing bonds' in J. Horten and M. Pyer (eds) *Children, Young People and Care*, London: Routledge, pp 158–174.

Evans, R. (2019) 'Interpreting family struggles in West Africa across majority–minority world boundaries: Tensions and possibilities', *Gender, Place & Culture*, 27(5), 717–732.

Evans, R. (2020) 'Picturing translocal youth: Self-portraits of young Syrian refugees and young people of African heritage in south-east England', *Population, Space & Place*, 26(6), e2303.

Evans, R. and Atim, A. (2011) 'Care, disability and HIV in Africa: Diverging or interconnected concepts and practices?', *Third World Quarterly*, 32(8), 1437–1454.

Evans, R. and Becker, S. (2009) *Children Caring for Parents with HIV and AIDS: Global Issues and Policy Responses*, Bristol: Policy Press.

Evans, R. and Becker, S. (2019) 'Comparing children's care work across majority and minority worlds' in A. Twum-Danso Imoh, M. Bourdillon and S. Meichsner (eds) *Global Childhoods Beyond the North-South Divide*, London: Palgrave Macmillan, pp 231–253.

Evans, R. and Thomas, F. (2009) 'Emotional interactions and an ethic of care: Caring relations in families affected by HIV and AIDS', *Emotions, Space and Society*, 2(2), 111–119.

Evans, R., Ribbens McCarthy, J., Bowlby, S., Wouango, J. and Kébé, F. (2016) 'Responses to death, care and family relations in urban Senegal', *Research Report 1*, Human Geography Research Cluster, University of Reading, http://blogs.reading.ac.uk/deathinthefamilyinsenegal/files/2016/02/Evans-et-al-2016-Report.pdf

Evans, R., Ribbens McCarthy, J., Bowlby, S., Wouango, J. and Kébé, F. (2017a) 'Producing emotionally sensed knowledge? Reflexivity and emotions in researching responses to death', *International Journal of Social Research Methodology*, 20(6), 585–598.

Evans, R., Ribbens McCarthy, J., Kébé, F., Bowlby, S. and Wouango, J. (2017b) 'Interpreting "grief" in Senegal: Language, emotions and cross-cultural translation in a Francophone African context', *Mortality*, 22(2), 118–135.

Evans, R., Bowlby, B., Gottzén, L. and Ribbens McCarthy, J. (2019) 'Unpacking "family troubles", care and relationality across time and space', *Children's Geographies*, 17(5), 501–513.

Ribbens McCarthy, J., Evans, R., Bowlby, S. and Wouango, J. (2018) 'Making sense of family deaths in urban Senegal: Diversities, contexts and comparisons', *Omega: Journal of Death and Dying*, 82(2), 230–260.

Romano, N., Mitchell, V. and Bozalek, V. (2019) 'Why walking the common is more than a walk in the park', *Journal of Public Pedagogies*, 4.

Ward, L. and Gahagan, B. (2010) 'Crossing the divide between theory and practice: Research and an ethic of care', *Ethics and Social Welfare*, 4(2), 210–216.

Zembylas, M., Bozalek, V. and Shefer, T. (2014) 'Tronto's notion of privileged irresponsibility and the reconceptualisation of care: Implications for critical pedagogies of emotion in higher education', *Gender and Education*, 26(3), 200–214.

# 5

# Research as praxis, interweaving a complex web

In this chapter, research with care is orientated as a praxis that involves people with various perspectives and knowledges. This chapter is about getting started on a research project, how to reach a decision about what to research, who may be involved in shaping that decision, and what influence this has on the design of a research project. As discussed in Chapter 1, people who get involved in research have a connection to the topic and a story about why that topic or issue is important to them. Those connections and stories change over time and exposure to being involved in research, and being involved in research can be a conduit for an evolving understanding of ourselves. Research interactions and relationships are dynamic and learning together is both a time of personal growth and possible exposure of vulnerabilities. To research together requires relational care and the space to get to know each other, time to build trust, space to talk and explore different ideas and make all sorts of connections, sometimes entirely unrelated to the topic. Attentiveness to the reasons that people are interested in the research gives a starting point to work from to understand what is important. Starting at the point of asking *what do you care about* or *what matters to you about this topic?* provides the space for that discussion. Asking people to talk about what they care about creates an open space for meaningful exchanges, a time for people to know what others are concerned about and how that relates to them personally and to gauge similarities and differences. What people would like to see as desired change in the world enables an understanding of priorities for action, however achievable they may be through research. In the conversations with researchers we spoke to for this book, we reflected on the origins of research projects and how they started. In this chapter we draw on the conversations we had with the people we spoke to – Bea, Bunty, Ceri, Ruth, Umut and Viv – about experiences of research partnerships and how this can be achieved with care.

## On research praxis

Research is praxis; a processual embodied cycle of judgement, action and reflection that constitutes experience and develops wisdom. Praxis is imbued with norms and customs which may or may not demonstrate care. To research with care, we advocate that researchers are attentive to marginalisation and inequality; respect the knowledge and experience that people bring and responsibly care for that contribution; work interdependently with people; care for the broader context in which the research sits as defined by the people who contribute; and undertake research that shows love for future generations of species and the planet. We advocate that experience is a fundamental building block of knowledge, and that individual and collective experiences are understood as intersectional, historically and temporally located, and situated in place. Following on from our critique of objectivity in Part I, we provide examples of the types of particularist knowledge Wynter (2003) called for, contextualised and complicated, as it inhabits life. To this end we offer an orientation of praxis that explicitly aims to be anti-racist after Gilroy et al (2019), that follows Wynter's humanness (Wynter, 2003) and that acknowledges the work of indigenous people on decolonising research (Smith, 1999/2012).

Tronto (2020) calls for advances in ethics of care that address inclusion and diversity. In research that values lived experience, recognition of whose voices lead and are present in research is critical to understand what contribution to knowledge is possible. Wynter (2003) suggests that what is needed to create connections and relations is *homo narrans* – the narratives of life shared through the stories people offer (Desai and Sanya, 2016). Rather than categorising people by role – researchers, research participants and experts by experience – we are people with inter-relatable stories. Being together, carefully listening and responding creates discovery, or deciphering, as Muñoz (1996) refers to research analytic interpretation, to collectively unpack and explore in order to gather insights about stories. And each story, each telling and each response makes visible the essence of the human and the multiplicity of positions and interpretations that are told. To achieve this unveiling of humanness is what Gilroy et al (2019) call convivial culture: 'very complicated forms of interdependence exist where one set of habits flows into others and all of them are altered by that encounter' (p 176). Wynter (2003) refers to praxis as humanness as it avails people of the opportunity to mix in genre-specific modes. People may not encounter what they consider *the other*, but still each person is interwoven in and with the other (Desai and Sanya, 2016, p 711). Care ethics research praxis is the embodiment of sharing together to disrupt and alter understanding to create new knowledge.

Telling stories is universal. Fiona Williams (2021) posits that telling stories about the future develops new possibilities for thinking together that provides hope for new action in much the same way that Haraway (2016) calls for imagined futures where humans and animals are intermeshed to save species from extinction. Part of praxis is to understand ourselves as positioned in the world and the assumptions that are brought to the discovery and deciphering of new knowledge. The knowledge brought by indigenous scholars is not well recognised in the philosophy of science debates, although the emphasis on human–non-human relations has been a constant in indigenous thought and knowledge (Rosiek et al, 2019). When people talk together, stories that appear to be unconnected turn out to be essential to new thinking. Linda Tuhiwai Smith (1999/2012) called for radical compassion through collaborations to imagine new decolonised possibilities. Decentring Eurocentrism and awareness of anti-racist practices, and seeking human connections (Kidd et al, 2020) supports progression towards Wynter's *homo narrans*. Desai and Sanya (2016, p 712) note that decolonial frameworks engender what Mignolo (2015) refers to as epistemic disobedience which calls for 'careful attention to the silences of Western epistemologies, the excavation of those silences and affirms the epistemic rights of the margins' (Desai and Sanya, 2016, p 712). The praxis orientation that fits with ethics of care thinking has at its core an aim of decolonising research, of anti-racist practice and of critically understanding humanness in relationships and relations with other species and the planet. Research praxis is about the processes of doing research together and the decisions that lead to actions, inactions and reactions, demonstrating responsibility and responding to others. We advocate that whatever type of research, there is a story about the research project that describes the origins, processes and practices of the work that draws out relationality and care.

## Getting started: what do we care about?

Sayer pointed out that people exercise moral judgements about what is right and wrong about the conditions that affect life for themselves and others. We suggest that a good place to start a conversation about what should be researched is to ask people what they care about. We have asked this question to groups in different settings. A group of researchers at the National Centre for Research Methods annual conference identified emergent ethical dilemmas in research projects that are not foreseen at the point of ethics committee agreement. Participants in research shared stories that were tangential to the research but were deeply troubling to the researchers who were unsure how to proceed with the divulgence. Researchers may find out a participant's motivation for being part of a project that sits outside of the remit of a project, or hear about difficult experiences. Participants at the conference discussed disappointment from participants that the research did not focus on a particular aspect, or challenges to the outcomes of the research because it would not make a material difference to their lives. Researchers discussed how managing relationships within the projects was emotional work that is often under-acknowledged and welcomed the opportunity to think through research with care in this way.

The second context in which we asked what people cared about was a group of service users and carers who work in partnership with academics in education and research (Patient/Public Involvement in Education and Research [PIER] at Bournemouth University). We spent a day with the group to discuss the preparation of a research network bid about broad societal challenges identified as key concerns to European citizens via the Eurobarometer in 2019 – ageing and care, climate emergency, democracy and migration. The day started with an outline of the ethics of care, and the participants were asked what they cared about. They identified homelessness, climate change, waste and other humans as their main concerns. Although the members of the group had known each other for quite some time, this meeting was asking them to do something they had not done before and there were discoveries and connections made within the group. The discussions were broad and, although time-limited, were wide-ranging and enabled people to talk about aspects of their selves and experiences not previously shared. These were captured by a cartoonist, Emma Paxton. We agreed that migration was a complex area where the concerns of the group could be seen together and the figure demonstrates the breadth of discussion and diverse connections that the group had around the issue (Figure 5.1).

Most of the care ethics contributors who we spoke to for this book identified a personal ontology that connects them with their topic of research. Doing research extended that personal connection through political and intellectual curiosity. They wanted to know more about their own experiences, how similar experiences affected others individually and collectively, and how experiences are theorised in academic discourses. Ruth's personal experiences growing up as a 'young carer' with a disabled parent and awareness of disabled people's rights was a key starting point for her research on young caregiving in the context of HIV (Evans and Becker, 2009). Ruth's research focus on families' experiences of care was initially prompted by personal experience as a 'young carer', and Ruth recounted how her personal connections continued to surface over the time she has been involved in researching care and bereavement in families. Over time and, in particular, by working reflexively with Jane Ribbens McCarthy, a sociologist and co-investigator, who inspired reflexive approaches designed to draw out those connections, Ruth's personal connection to the research became clearer to her. In one research project, the researchers interviewed each other and Ruth was surprised at her emotionally intense reaction when discussing the death of a family member. Through this experience, Ruth understood herself and her own experiences in a new light (Evans et al, 2017a). The reflexive approach adopted in the team opened up dialogues about minority and majority world perspectives on 'bereavement'. The researchers aimed to draw out and explore differences and commonalities in experiences and approaches researchers may share with research participants

**Figure 5.1:** Discussing care: migration

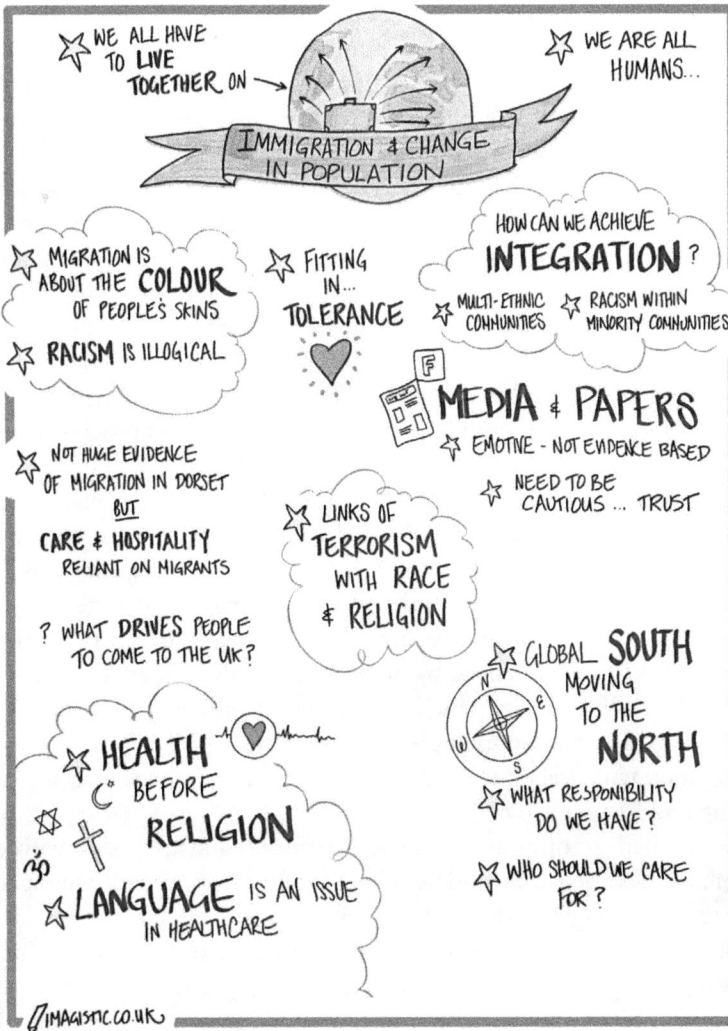

Source: Emma Paxton, Imagistic.co.uk

across socioeconomic and cultural boundaries (Ribbens McCarthy et al, 2018; Evans, 2019). Ceri initially focused on the natural sciences before reconnecting with her interest in participative democracy through her PhD study (Davies, 2016), exploring practices of activism, participation and social movements in theory and in practice as a volunteer. Ceri's experience of community activism and union activism within her family from the Welsh valleys was eventually reflected in her engagement in qualitative research with a strong deliberative and political flavour. As a student, Umut noted how the ideas of migration and citizenship were separated, contrary to her personal experience as a migrant and an important prompt to investigate migrant women's experiences of citizenship (Erel, 2018; Erel et al, 2018). We asked Umut about her own experiences of migration and she explained that she had moved as a young child from Turkey to Germany, where people from Turkey were excluded and oppressed. The policy term used in Germany at the time of reunification was 'enmity to foreigners', and the idea was promoted by the state that racism did not exist in Germany, however, an era of increased racist attacks highlighted the experience of racism towards migrants who were seen as 'foreigners' despite having lived in Germany for many years or even decades. Umut's family saw themselves as cosmopolitan citizens who were part of German society, but German society saw them very differently. These experiences and intellectual curiosity seeded the ideas for research into citizenship and migration. Viv initially practised as a social worker, continued her commitment to democratisation of process (Bozalek and Zembylas, 2017), and social justice through critical pedagogies (Zembylas et al, 2014). Viv has sought innovations through the application of feminist ethico-onto-epistemologies in her work with academics and students to create new ways of relational knowledge production. Her emphasis is on the interdependence of beings and things in understanding differently, and the processes by which inter-relational transformations can be achieved. Her work has been influenced by Selma Sevenhuijsen, Joan Tronto, Karen Barad and Donna Haraway, which has brought together care and diffractive methodologies that value multiple ways of knowing. Viv's work is often in collaboration with academics to develop new understanding about teaching, learning and knowledge creation.

Bea also had a commitment to social justice and getting involved in research enabled Bea to extend her concerns for the welfare of older people and activism through an ethics of care lens (Barnes et al, 2018). Bea saw the potential for research to identify the normative discourse about wellbeing that was present in policy and strategy documents, but missing in funding and policy objectives and therefore what was possible in practice. This situated knowledge contributed an important element of understanding about the difference in policy rhetoric and the experience of older people, an important contribution to research. Inclusion in the research provided a platform for formal and legitimate critical perspectives on policy and practice. Working alongside Bea and Marian, Bunty gave some very precious time towards the end of her life to examine care for older people. Bunty initially got involved with Age UK to get to know people when she was new to the area, and volunteered to be part of the research group with Bea. Bunty wanted something meaningful to do and was tired of unfulfilled promises by governments. Bunty was always interested in other people's points of view. Initially hesitant, she had never done research before and thought it would be good to be part of something different. Bunty talked about the welfare state claiming to offer security for older people and how that broken promise had been a political motivation for involvement in the research. As I, Marian, reflected on these questions about the relationship between what I researched and what matters to me, I suggested that generalised social justice concerns had coalesced around issues that increasingly connected to family and personal experiences of mental health, ageing and care. My discovery of feminist care ethics came at a point in my life when I was trying to reconcile my reactions to the personal experience of my mother's dementia, with the impact of having researched political campaigning by disability organisations. Disability rights claims based in justice ethics and citizenship seemed inadequate to address what was necessary to enable mum to live in the world as well as possible with her dementia. Discovering Sevenhuijsen's (1998) book, *Citizenship and the Ethics of Care: Feminist Considerations of Justice, Morality and Politics*, offered a way of reconciling care with citizenship. The ethics of care offered me a way of thinking and doing that made sense personally, politically and intellectually.

I, Tula, have family experiences of mental health challenges and practised as a mental health nurse. Like many other mental health workers, I saw the injustices of the system through the harms that people experienced within it, and empathised strongly with the aims of the mental health survivor movement to promote recovery through anti-oppressive practice (Brannelly, 2011, 2016), considered in practice using ethics of care. When I migrated to Aotearoa New Zealand, I used the ethics of care to guide research practices in partnership with Māori (Brannelly and Boulton, 2017; Brannelly, 2018). I grew up in a large Irish family in Birmingham, UK, embedded in an Irish community. There are so many people of similar heritage that the term Birmingham Irish is a subculture in the city. Growing up in the 1970s and 1980s, the Irish were disliked, especially when the Irish Republican Army were active. The dominant narrative among the Irish was one of colonisation: how the British had exploited the people; stolen the land; tried to destroy the culture; banned the language; and how people were disadvantaged and displaced through poverty. This background positioned me as sympathetic to the struggles of Māori to the consequences of living with colonisation, and to the experiences of mental health challenges as a rational reaction to a difficult life.

The seed for a research project is often inspired through an interplay of intellectual and personal situated knowledges, through conversations, reading and hearing others' experiences. In our conversation, Viv offered important insights about the value of talking time to read others' work, to understand it for what it is, questioning ideas from different disciplinary positions and reading work through other theorists as part of response-ability (Bozalek and Zembylas, 2017). Ideas for research rarely come from an isolated and distanced position, contrary to the portrayal of academics as lone thinkers and actors. Research ideas come from an immersion in the world and discussions with other people. Early conversations about a research idea are a temperature gauge of the importance and relevance of the idea, and whether it resonates with the voice of experience. Where that spark happens, the research journey begins. Bea described knowing the research 'inside and out' – a reference to embodied knowledge meshed with intellectual understanding about researching care for older people. Bea knew a lot from her professional involvement with the experience of ageing – an experience that had given her a close understanding of how this is experienced by older people. At the start she didn't 'know about' care ethics, but quickly recognised this as a way of making sense of many things that both troubled and inspired her. Bea's coming together with Marian and Lizzie enabled that lightbulb moment. Commitment to pursuing the research idea comes through the acid test of experience, whether the newly conceptualised idea makes sense in the world.

Taking care with people means not creating a hierarchy of knowledge by valuing some contributions over others, or inadvertently demeaning some experiences as having less value. As research is about a stated thing, it is usual to request only knowledge that is associated to the identified phenomena, rather than the interpreted knowledge of the person in their intersectional, multiple roles. Brown (2018), a psychotherapist and academic, gives the example in mental health research where some people who contribute do so from a position of experience, but everyone has experiences of mental health and challenges through everyday life experiences. Brown prefers a continuum of mental health and distress in this context, moving away from the need for formal diagnostic criteria so often rejected by people who receive them. Adopting precise criteria for inclusion in a research project can be problematic as it may exclude or repel some people who would be very helpful in building new understandings. A good example is the use of stigmatised terms such as dementia or schizophrenia, disliked by people who are affected, who would prefer to be identified as having memory issues or psychosis, or by the name of the illness, such as Alzheimer's. And denoting a characteristic by which people are legitimated to contribute signals to people that this one aspect of their identity is prioritised, thereby missing the chance to share other aspects of their lives and experiences that can help understanding. Sensitivity to multiple perspectives is possible when people get to know each other. This was evident in the Older People and Wellbeing Project. We (the researchers) invited people to take part as co-researchers on the basis that they knew about being old. But being old means a lifetime of experience and among this group were people who had worked in health and social care settings, who had experience of activism in other contexts and who had administrative and legal skills. This is evident in the brief portraits of Bunty and Liz in the introduction to this part of the book. To disregard these was neither respectful nor helpful, but Marian reflected on the need to learn about this and what it meant both for what co-researchers brought to the project and how they responded to the experience of being asked to take part because of their age (Barnes et al, 2018).

In our research, when we have introduced the ethics of care to people who do not know about it, there has usually been an instant understanding of how important care is to us as interdependent beings. People see care as something that has been hiding in plain sight, so crucial to our lives, ubiquitous yet too often unnamed or understated. By starting out by being attentive to what people care about it is more possible to create careful research practices and to take care not to (re)enact any trauma through research. It demonstrates that starting out together is a new undertaking that is unknown but discoverable, and capable of generating new knowledge together.

Being part of research is about creating new understandings through new experiences, and with it an emerging reality for everyone involved. At the start of research projects, initial conversations can be intense as people share their experiences and perspectives about the topic. There is often a steep learning curve as people inform each other of their perspectives. Tentacles reach out into places that were not envisaged, new links are made to other ideas and experiences. These conversations can help (re)interpret experiences through exposure to new intellectual and experiential knowledge. New understandings can help us heal, can shine a new light on a long-standing idea to change how we see the world. The transformational journey starts with these conversations that enlighten us, which Marian reflected on as *a journey not entirely of your making,* such are the external influences on it. Marian reflected on Bea's conversation and made the connection with Gilligan's work uncovering subjugated voices. We keep going back to the idea of voices that are seldom heard, with women's voices surprisingly needing to be surfaced. In my (Tula's) research, learning from people with experience has influenced every project, usually at a fundamental level. Developing an app with people who use mental health crisis services, I immediately understood very differently the experience of a crisis as a drawn out, long period of distress over weeks, rather than a short-term peak of distress over hours. This has a fundamental impact on the conceptualisation of what might help in that situation. Being challenged by disability activists when rooms on campus were inaccessible was fundamental to understanding the built environment. The sense of panic when travelling with a mobility disabled researcher because the train journey was altered, was an experiential understanding I had never had before. These exposures are minimal in comparison to the everyday difficulties that co-researchers faced, and demonstrate the importance of including experiential knowledge.

Personal experiences may become exposed or emerge as part of our identities as researchers. Ruth discussed how she had over time come to recognise her own trauma through coming closer to research participants' experiences of trauma. Originally designed as a therapeutic tool, Ruth adapted body mapping for her research, which involved drawing a life-size outline of the self and mapping onto the body different aspects of identity, personal life history, embodied experiences, care and support. Some time later Ruth realised she had represented herself in a particular way through this exercise, omitting important aspects of her identity and experiences of trauma. The powerful emotional experience and representations produced made her think about the importance of creating a safe space to hold the potential distress of participants and, while it may be therapeutic, there is a need to consider carefully whether, how and when to use the approach in the future. Learning through research is expected, but we are highlighting that it is also sometimes unexpected, unpredictable, insightful and surprising. Ceri reflected on this as a question of relativism, where some learning can be predicted but personal growth is dependent on the foundations on which it sits. Sometimes you hit a nerve, your reaction is a surprise. Reflection and unpacking can bring fruitful insights, reading experience through a theoretical perspective, or isolating an example to explore in depth through multiple readings. In Chapter 2 we discussed Sayer's position on post-disciplinary approaches that value multiplicity in drawing out broad and what can appear unconnected understandings to explore and expand an idea to reach into its extremities and see where it takes you. In the initial stages of research, muddling experience, knowledge and exploration illuminates this approach in research practice. There is an intention to draw out interconnectedness about ecologies, environments, realities and possibilities, to be broad and expansive. In ethics of care research this is an ethical necessity to surface voices that may not be heard, draw out those connections that otherwise remain unknown and a relational imperative to value the speakers and contributions.

## Getting started together in research with care

Participatory methodologists (who may have lived experience) ask people with experience to contribute to research. This happens in one of three ways. There may be long-standing relationships with groups that are established to do research projects who then continue to identify new research and a cycle of bidding and completion of projects. The group work together to identify topics and the research is co-produced. Alternatively, researchers may identify the topic and then ask people who are directly affected to contribute to the development of a bid and subsequent research. This is researcher-led and develops the research initially in consultation with greater involvement over time. The researcher may build capacity with the group and work towards a longer relationship. Or, a researcher may ask for involvement in response to a funding call and take a semi-developed bid to people with experience for discussion with a view to continuing involvement if the proposal is funded. We (Marian and Tula), and the people we spoke to for the book, have experience of all three approaches at getting started in research. We argue that unless care is practised, the relationship is unlikely to endure the length of the project.

Marian, Bea and Bunty were part of a long-term relationship between the university and Age UK, together with Lizzie Ward. Marian and Bea found a synthesis between the aims of the organisation and the approach taken with the research. The wellbeing project was a new evolution in exploring what care meant to older people. It was Bea's first introduction to the ethics of care, which she described as a wonderful fit with personal values – a 'synchronicity'. I (Marian) have noted that the ethics of care offers a language to talk about something that can be difficult to talk about, so there is a sense of lifting the lid on something that had been suppressed or inadequately articulated. In the early days of this project, after the initial ideas had been discussed, I gave a 'seminar' on care ethics to the research team of older co-researchers. This prompted an immediate recognition that it 'made sense', that this was an obvious way of thinking about people, their relationships with each other and with the world. This reflected experience in another context. I had been involved in deliberative discussions with older people about 'what human rights mean to you'. This highlighted the discomfort many felt about the individual focus of a rights approach. The discussants returned repeatedly to the importance of thinking about how their actions impacted on others and on their relationships with them, rather than solely thinking about their rights as individuals. Gilligan's articulation of the ethics of care was based in research with young people struggling to work out what is the right thing to do in different situations. The different voice she heard was one that prioritised relationships and responsibilities rather than rights and rules. Research by Fiona Williams and colleagues, which included exploring decision making among women with young children about how best to care for them, similarly demonstrated the relational nature of moral agency (Williams, 2004). Our work with old people indicates that relational ethics continue to characterise the way in which people seek to make sense of how to live well throughout their lives.

For Bea, the ethics of care project came at a time when she was hanging on in a changed organisational environment where she no longer felt her values were being put into practice. Being involved in the research gave her an anchor. The commitment to hearing the voices of the most marginalised was very meaningful. Bea interviewed people responding to an advert from Age UK inviting people to get involved as co-researchers in the project – the aim was to make this process as informal as possible. Bunty was one of the volunteers who responded to the advert and said going for this interview with Bea was one of the most scary things in her life. Bunty felt intimidated by intelligent people and the thought of the interview scared her. It is worth noting that people are intimidated by the idea that they could get involved with research – the idea may be very appealing, but the thought of getting involved may be challenging for many people. Care is needed to make getting involved as easy as possible, considering the venue, who is present and how hospitable the event is.

Ruth reflected on the challenge of approaching an organisation at short notice to contribute to research proposals and managing expectations, especially given the highly competitive nature of social science funding. Some of Ruth's research has been with refugees, and the organisations are short of time and resources. She found it crucial to develop ongoing relationships of trust with key practitioners, for example through wider citizenship/voluntary roles such as University of Sanctuary work to welcome sanctuary seekers at the university, being a trustee for organisations, and developing research ideas based on exploratory pilot research with families and informal conversations with practitioners and policy makers which inform larger grant applications, rather than expecting people to contribute directly to written research proposals which may not be successful. Getting started meant listening carefully to the people in the organisation to understand what matters to them and incorporating those ideas into the proposal, or future proposals. Umut also talked about listening carefully to one of the organisations she worked with to explore the kinds of opportunities and ways of working that appealed to the group. Umut worked with some groups who were pre-established: for example, the group who were connected to the project that examined motherhood and citizenship knew each other. But even when people do know each other Umut noted the need for hospitality and time to build trust for the group to accept the researchers. More marginalised groups often needed more time to coalesce, and she and the research team designed workshops sensitively to generate trust and develop a shared language that was acceptable to all those involved. In the No Recourse to Public Funds group Umut noted an initial reluctance to share information, although the group slowly thawed to each other. People were sometimes socially isolated and that took a while to lift, but then great support networks were developed independently of the research team. Over time, some people had long-term involvement in several projects and projects built on each other, and the women were invited to present to other community groups for example.

Both Tula and Marian also reflected on their experiences of approaching user and community groups to take part in research and being met with a sense of suspicion or guardedness. We both recognised an unwillingness to become involved. Tula had a recent experience of trying to negotiate a discussion about involvement in research with a local mental health group, but over a succession of meetings realised that the group were opposed to participating. Community groups sometimes need to be exclusive to protect themselves from exploitation – they may well have had experience of being asked to contribute in ways which have not suited their way of working. Researchers may be approaching groups after they have had a challenging experience and the timing may not be right, or they may approach in a way that the group are sensitive to and that echo previous negative experiences. Researchers approaching community groups are likely to meet a range of responses and being attentive to them can start a discussion about the willingness or otherwise of involvement.

I (Tula) have spent time with people with experience in university and non-governmental organisation settings to build capacity for involvement in research. SureSearch at the University of Birmingham had a sub-group who were interested in knowing more about methods and doing research, and we spent a few days together to understand methods and approaches and to garner research ideas. One non-governmental organisation in Wellington, New Zealand was mental health user led, and had a youth governance group who were consulted by government on policy and practice changes. Of the broader group, four were interested in getting involved and came along to the university for a two-day introduction to research, which focused on a funded project. Three of the young people worked as peer researchers and designed the interview schedule, interviewed young people, participated in the analysis of the project and dissemination. One decided the role was not for them as they did not want to remain immersed in thinking about mental health and service use and decided on a change of focus. Offering a session to PIER at Bournemouth University more recently, the emphasis was on previous experiences as peer researchers and how they evaluated that involvement. People with experience wanted to be involved in research but wanted to be taken seriously and for their ideas to influence the research, which was not always their experience. The discussion was about how to assess a researcher for their ability to enable good participation. People who are curious about involvement would like to be offered the opportunity to be involved without responsibility to see if it is something that they could take on, such as shadowing in a project to see if they could take on the responsibility and cope with the work. We advocate that researchers are attentive to the group and their situation and understand the everyday challenges that people face in getting involved. Peer to peer support often helps people settle into groups and facilitating involvement that does not allow dominance within a group is necessary for people to stay involved and be valued.

## Achieving epistemic justice from the start

One way of working well with people in research is to think through how to support involvement prior to starting to work with the group. Careful consideration is needed to invite people in. Who are the people who will be contributing, what is their collective story, what narrative is their story part of? What am I asking them to do and say and how does this connect to broader questions that are of concern to their people or community? How have these questions been asked in the past, and by whom? How competent am I in asking this of the group, and how confident do I feel about this? Do I need help to do this well? In research guided by an ethics of care, it is necessary to be aware of and evaluate the possibilities of presenting research in a way that avoids or addresses invalidation, discreditation or the silencing of voices. While listening is obvious, and not listening is likely to be unintended on the part of researchers, it is too commonly experienced by some communities (Edwards et al, 2020). Even when we listen, it may take some time before we really hear.

Edwards et al (2020) brought together indigenous and non-indigenous researchers to help researchers from the global north in their approach to working with indigenous communities. Research in the present is influenced by the past, and that past may harbour historical injustices carried with people in the present (Smith, 2014). The framing of the issue is the first step in making clear the assumptions that underpin research and has implications for the involvement of communities. Preparation includes negotiating with people from that community who vouch for you as a reliable, non-offensive person who is not likely to do any harm. As Edwards et al (2020, p 3049) state: 'Indigenous research, though, aspires to critical, transformative and to benefit the community or collective grouping as they define that themselves. Western dominated research is often challenged as being deficit based, identifying needs and risks, and attempting to solve social problems that are identified as challenges by governments.'

Epistemic injustice in the framing and conceptualisation of research positions people/communities as unable to come up with solutions to the challenges they face, inadequate explanation of the systems that are complicit in the situation being upheld, and denying the reality of the lived experience. Coming together to do research carries with it a responsibility to forge futures where these harms are not repeated and may be repaired. To do so, a political awareness of the position of the group who are approached to be involved in research is needed, and this understanding becomes deepened and more nuanced as the group works together. We advocate that researchers go in with their eyes open to these possibilities and have thought about how to receive this kind of knowledge that may be new to them. Competent approaches include discussions with people to understand what concerns them about getting involved in research, practices such as careful listening through open discursive spaces to share that knowledge and its impact. The researchers who contributed to this book noted the problematic dominant narratives commonly circulated, for instance in government policy and the media, that made people cautious about talking about their experiences. In the UK, Umut noted that Muslim women were not viewed only as mothers who cared, but as a threat to social cohesion and the security of the nation (Erel et al, 2018). Any echo of this positioning will have the effect of silencing these women.

Ceri reflected on her research examining university and community partnerships where the contrast between Canada and the UK was stark. In Canada a partnership week of activities with First Nations peoples meant that Ceri immediately saw a very different way of thinking about and enacting relationality where people and place were considered together and ancestors were present in the conversation. This made Ceri think differently about how researchers introduce themselves, and she changed written in-person introductions that included personal statements about herself and the story of why the research was important to her. Reciprocity was foregrounded and Ceri was mindful of what constituted a gift; she offered practical help to the community such as helping with catering or cleaning up. There was less emphasis on professional relationship boundaries and people quickly described themselves as friends. Care was explicit and expected. This reflects other indigenous contexts. In Māori *tikanga* (custom), the new endeavour will strengthen the links and build support and respect on both sides (*mana*), and this is set out formally through protocol. If there has been some misdemeanour in the past, the new relationship will set out to repair and renew that, a fresh start with acknowledgement of the pain of the past. In western cultures we do not dig this deep into links, or act this formally though ceremony. In *Te Ara Tika* (Māori ethical framework for research) Hudson et al (2010) suggest that research starts with the concept of *Kia Tūpato* (to be careful) to consider the potential benefit of a research project. *Kia āta-whakaaro* (precise analysis) and *kia āta-korero* (robust discussion) of the practical/ethical/spiritual dimensions of the project is necessary to provide a foundation to *kia āta-whiriwhiri* (consciously determine) the conditions which allow the project to *kia āta-haere* (proceed with understanding). Taking care of the people, acceptability of the research to the community and that the research empowers the community are central concerns *to Te Ara Tika* before research begins (Hudson et al, 2010). We think this is consistent with what we are advocating to research with care.

## Conclusion

The ethics of care is a way of thinking about research. As such it is a lens to view the systems present in the everyday world. When I (Tula) worked in the bicultural context of Aotearoa New Zealand and trying to avoid causing any offence to indigenous partners, it was to the ethics of care that I turned for guidance as it offered a way of thinking through the process with care, and how to prepare myself to do that. Viv talked in our conversation about how she 'thought with' the ethics of care ever since she knew about it. It has the advantage that it can be used to plan how to frame research, create hospitable events that give people the opportunity to talk and be together. Caring about how we research creates the space that researchers need to give the time and attention to it so that the research starts as it means to go on, aims to understand what people care about, how it affects them, the harms that may be associated with experiences, and the emotional work that people carry with them and generously contribute. Becoming involved in research is an emergent experience, and one in which people expect to respond to, not always in a way that is anticipated. We are all in that together and all have something to contribute to that process. In the next chapter we turn to the doing of research to focus on how an ethics of care informs our thinking about the inextricable interdependencies of doing research.

# 6

# Doing research together: interdependencies to maintain, sustain and renew our worlds

This chapter applies ethics of care to the process of *doing* research. We draw on experiential knowledge to tell the stories shared with us by the people we spoke to for this book about research projects guided by, and reflected on, using the ethics of care. During research projects, unpredictable situations can arise that may require revisions to the research plan, challenge the fundamental assumptions that inform the research, or uncover more significant situations that require attention. Changes to the project may be externally influenced, for example by ethics committees or other governance groups requesting alterations to the research. More personal reactions to the research also occur, and attention to this experience influences how the research is practised, and how to care for the people involved. At each turn, a response is needed that builds trust and solidarity, and makes space for reflexivity. In the last chapter we discussed getting started on research projects and in the next chapter we discuss the later stages of research – analysis, dissemination and endings; this chapter is about refining the project, collecting data, initial reactions and observations, and working these through together.

There are two parts to this chapter. The first is about how the process of doing the research is as important as the outcomes and, indeed, itself produces what we might think of as either outcomes or legacies of the research. We discuss how the ethics of care has guided these processes of research, and the sorts of thinking used to traverse the situated complexities we are likely to encounter. The second part is about caring for the people involved, and how to engage care for people in research projects they take part in. We discuss how entanglements, or inextricable interdependencies (Kittay, 2015), produce insightful moments of knowledge, and that this is only possible when good relationships are sustained, and sometimes repaired when we work together in research projects. We reflect on what to do when things are not going well, and how to avoid relationships being jeopardised. This is not to say that people stay in research projects at all costs, but that the decisions about whether to continue or leave the research are made together with care and responsibility to each other. Caring for the people involved in the research also applies to people who we are in contact with in the broader academic arena. We reflect on the roles of those who are not directly involved in doing the research projects, but are connected to them by, for example, reviewing funding grant proposals or journal articles arising from projects. We suggest how the ethics of care can also guide a collaborative and supportive approach to these influential practices.

One part of doing research together is having competence to do the work. As we have suggested previously, competence can develop during the course of doing research and we need to recognise the value of what we have called the 'distributed competence' of different members of the team. Competence is also knowing limitations, and seeking help when it is needed. In this chapter we expand on working with people with experience throughout the process of collecting data, drawing on how people who come together to research have used the ethics of care in order to navigate research relationships that will encourage and support participation. People with experience who have experience of being involved in research projects talk about whether the academic researchers 'get it' or not. This means that the researchers understand the value of experiential knowledge and enable people to influence the research through competent inclusion, listening and facilitation. Researchers who don't 'get it' have already decided the shape of the project, and consequently offer people with experience a narrow and defined role. In contrast, if innovative ways of engaging people in the team and in the research more broadly are shared, there is potential for surprise, growth and learning for all those involved.

In the conversations we had with the people who contributed to the book, we provided these questions in advance of our conversations in order to encourage reflection about what care in research looks like, and what worked and what didn't in the research they had undertaken:

- What are the relationships like in the team? Here we are interested primarily in relationships among those carrying out the work, those who were the participants of the research, those who commissioned or funded it and others who had any interest or role within it.
- Thinking about Tronto's phases of care and the principles associated with them: what was required in terms of attentiveness to others during the course of the project? How was responsibility exercised and by whom? Who did you feel accountable to? What different kinds of competence came into play during the project and did the process enable competence to develop? How did people respond to taking part? Was there any evidence of building solidarity during the course of the work? What dilemmas did you experience with respect to the relational aspects of research?

The responses to these questions and our reflections were themed into the two areas of discussion that came through strongly in our conversations, and it is to these that we now turn – the process of doing research and taking care of people as we do so. We discuss the kinds of practices that we and others have used in research projects that have been particularly successful in getting the research done in a way that ensures care for the people involved. The people we spoke to for this book reflected on their experiences working with people from various and diverse communities and what worked well in different contexts. An intrinsic part of the care work was knowing the people involved and continuing to provide a space where people can lead discussions or contact others in the team for support.

## The importance of the process

A clear theme that ran throughout our conversations was that the process of doing the research was as important as the outcome in terms of research findings. Doing research together creates a space in which the convivial culture of sharing can influence each other's thinking. This is the transformational space where illuminating discussions can happen. The people we spoke to talked about understanding things differently – both about themselves and other people, their perceptions and experiences. The exchanges they had with others involved were not always easy and could be quite confrontational, people needed time to reflect, so how the conversations were facilitated really mattered. Despite these experiences of illuminating discussions, the transformations that occur, and how these come about, these stories of the process of research are not often shared. They are not seen to constitute 'outcomes' to be reported to commissioners in order to support recommendations for policy. Viv has called for a shift from the focus on the academic artefact, be it a report or article, to a critical telling of the method by which the artefact came into being.

Telling the story with a critical lens is important because there are normative research processes that fit some communities and groups better than others, and unsurprisingly, dominant communities are better served. So, attention is needed to draw out positionality, assumptions that change, who is involved and what that means for knowledge development. Viv gave the example of a collaborative walking group where academics came together with the intention of creating a space for interdisciplinary discussions (Romano et al, 2019). In the article, Viv and her colleagues identify a long-term relationship where, in a coffee shop, overlooking a green space, the collaborators had shared ideas over coffee and food, until they decided to walk and talk around the common. This surfaced new conversations, ideas and understanding about interpreting privilege in post-apartheid South Africa.

We felt an exchange of affect between those present, the ghosts of colonial and apartheid histories, and the implications for our ongoing teaching.

> Following Haraway's (2016) 'staying with the trouble' and Tsing et al.'s (2017) 'how to live on a damaged planet', the relationships between human and non-human continue to haunt us, as we grapple with the im/possibility of finding common ground in a country devastated by colonial and apartheid violences. (Romano et al, 2019, p 235)

The setting was provocative to the discussion by connecting the people to the land and places of oppression and gain. For me (Tula), this was allied with asking people to understand their colonisation story when working in settler and indigenous communities to support decolonising practice. Everyone in Aotearoa New Zealand, for example, has a colonial story. Knowing how historical actions are reproduced and re-enacted in the present, how that influences how we are positioned and therefore relate to each other, helps people to acknowledge and understand their position in relation to others. Starting with whose land you are on is a grounded acknowledgement to get started on the process. In research, this asks us to identify who we are in the making of knowledge in order to relate to each other.

Viv has continued to think through social work practice with the ethics of care and how students may learn best to understand the position of the other to enhance relational social work skills. She emphasises the significance of responsibility in order to consider the roles that social work and other helping professions have had in generating past harms. Professions enact societal customs and norms and are associated with some horrific occurrences that have been practised in the name of care. Among practices that are clearly not care is the role of social work and its complicity in assimilation policies that removed Black children from their families to place them with White families. In colonised countries, anti-indigenous racist policies are enacted through state actors, including nurses, social workers and the police. Viv has written about the need for recognition for such actions to achieve 'justice-to-come' (Bozalek et al, 2021). Professional groups, such as social workers and nurses, who consider their responsibility to the communities in which they work and acknowledge the harms of the past, demonstrate the ability to learn from the past for a different future.

In the previous chapter we focused on the way in which research is framed at the start of the process. But this is something that needs to be continually revisited during projects. Umut talked about the care that needs to be taken about the acceptability of the framing and language used so that people who have been marginalised start to trust the team and feel able to contribute. In her research, demonstrating a critical approach to the policy that disadvantages the women negotiating their lives as migrants communicated a clear indicator of sensitivity to the position that they are in. What was needed in this situation was recognition of the women and what was important to them so that the affirmation built trust. In Erel et al (2017), Umut and her colleagues discuss how they used participatory theatre to enable migrant mothers to express acts of citizenship, and how the theatre became rehearsals for sociopolitical transformations. Theatre enabled participants to articulate subjugated identities and challenge pathologising discourses of migrant mothers as outside of citizenship. The timing of this work coincided with the political positioning of Muslims in Britain as unwelcome unless able to learn English and engage on British values and culture (Erel et al, 2018). In the research, participants told their stories of mothering as an act of citizenship and these were played out by professional actors which enabled representations of self that participants found more useful. The researchers highlight that some of them shared some aspects of social location (as migrants or first generation themselves), but it was also their political values that influenced their broad research question: 'What is it like to be a migrant mother?'. This created the conditions in which these women were able to flourish as the research was a stark contrast to exclusionary practices experienced in other contexts. Rather than basing the research on interviews that carried the danger of replicating experiences of interviews associated with asylum or refugee processes where the implications of answers were far-reaching, the process of enacting what was important to them reduced unease and supported participation in the research.

Another project that Umut led explored migrants' access to social security and social services (Erel et al, 2017). During the workshops hosted for this project, a group that had been in the UK for many years challenged being described as 'migrants' and asked that the term be reconsidered. The people in the group saw themselves as citizens who had a right to be in the UK. Umut recounted that the women, who were mostly African and Caribbean, identified that they had worked in the UK, most had been in the UK for 11–24 years, and were part of the UK. While the group were referred to as migrants in a policy context, and this was considered an acceptable term for policy makers, funders and ethics committees, it was not acceptable to the people directly affected. That conversation had an impact on the language used in the study and a short play created to communicate findings was renamed to reflect the women's wishes. Tula had encountered similar experiences when doing research with people with dementia who viewed the term dementia as derogatory and wanted to be referred to using a diagnostic term, such as living with Alzheimer's Disease, or a less stigmatised term such as memory loss. These are the conversations that move the discussion forward about acceptability and discriminatory terms that eventually might need to be rejected in order to reflect what matters to those involved.

We (Tula and Marian) both have experiences of ways in which careful researching with others requires an attentiveness that can change the way we go about things. The impact of having young co-researchers involved and the importance of the partnership with Māori were crucial in the evaluation of the alcohol and drug service that I (Tula) led (Brannelly et al, 2013b). Three young people worked as co-researchers to interview the young people, while I and other researchers interviewed the parents, school provider and the police. In one interview, Josh, a young Māori man with experience of mental health challenges and I went to do an interview with a young Māori man and his mum. When Josh and I arrived at the house, there were many of the *whānau* (extended family) present, all of whom wanted to have their say about what had happened. Abandoning the idea of individual interviews, all the participants were included. The young person and mum were asked for consent and were surprised that this was requested on an individual basis. Josh held the interview in the kitchen with five or six siblings and cousins, and I talked to a further six people in the lounge. The situation was joyful as the *whānau* stated their love and support for the *rangatahi* (young person), the misadventures were recounted and commented on, the *rangatahi* listened and was embarrassed when the examples of his behaviours were shared, and finally the *whānau* discussed a way forward. In another interview, a co-researcher, Jess, interviewed a 13-year-old who had been sleeping in abandoned buildings with a group of older homeless people. The girl had been drinking alcohol and taking drugs with the group and her parents were very concerned for her wellbeing. Jess introduced herself, and for the first 20 minutes of the recorded interview talked about cats, eventually getting a response and starting a broader conversation. The interview was remarkable for the candid way in which the girl described her life on the streets in comparison to her life at home, how she felt more accepted out of home than at home. On listening to the recording, it was clear that unless this was another young person with experience who was able to share feelings of not belonging and intense emotional response, this story would never be heard. These were two really important interviews for the evaluation of the service, they provided quality data and influenced the thinking of the team about the provision of the service. But the stories of how this data was achieved were not told in the report or elsewhere, and remained untold until now, only acknowledged within the team.

Reflecting on the process of researching older people and wellbeing, Bunty also spoke about the way people responded to the invitation to take part in interviews. Not only were most pleased to be interviewed because of potential benefits of the research to other older people, they also valued being asked to talk about things they had never been asked about before; these things mattered to them, but no one had previously indicated this kind of interest. The old people who were interviewed experienced personal recognition and a sense of building solidarity with other old people even though they may never meet again. Telling the story of the process, a narrative of the events and pivotal moments that influenced how new knowledge was created, surfaces how the research process itself generated learning about what can generate wellbeing. How we carried out the wellbeing project both contributed to wellbeing and enabled learning about what it is that generates this (Barnes et al, 2018).

In the conversations with the people we spoke to for this part of the book, we reflected on the kinds of changes that we made to ensure that our approach was acceptable to the different communities with which we have worked. Ceri reflected on her time in Uganda as a postgraduate student, where among other things, she learnt to 'check herself' to prepare how to frame a conversation, and how to describe people without using racialised terms. To enable better participation with Māori, I (Tula) took a language course in *te reo* Māori to improve pronunciation, and to learn how to introduce myself (*mihi* that signals where you are from and who you are connected to) formally in a *powhiri* (a formal greeting and welcome). Knowing when to stand forward and fulfil your role, and when to fall back to learn from others was itself a demonstration of competence. I was unknown to the people providing services, which is common when evaluating or researching health and social services and needed to establish quickly that I was someone who could be trusted, despite my shortcomings in language and knowledge of *tikanga* (customs). Throughout the project, the Māori people in the project were generous in their acceptance and guidance.

Both I (Tula) and Ceri spoke about really thinking things through as anticipatory preparation intended to fully consider the context to be able to respond well. Attentiveness is necessary throughout the process of doing research as the way in which participants respond to the process requires us to make adjustments to our practices. Careful preparation was described by Ceri who gave the example of the Citizens' Assembly, which is a meeting arranged with citizens to discuss an important issue, such as migration or climate emergency. Because the issue is important to people, something that they care deeply about, care is needed to really think through how the issue is presented, what people are being asked to do, and the way in which they are likely to respond to this. The process can include asking people to listen to and engage in troubling stories. Researchers need to think about how to provide that information in a way that enables people to engage and respond, but also to be aware of responses they may not have anticipated. Ceri talked about offering a glossary of language with notes about how the terms may be contested and why they are used in specific circumstances. As we have seen from Umut's experience, language and terminology frame the topic, but also help people to understand what terms are acceptable and why they are used. In some cases the contested nature of language is part of what the research aims to explore and being attentive to the way in which people respond to its use helps us understand what they care about and why. As a facilitator in the meetings, Ceri talked about the need for attentiveness throughout the meeting, to read the room, scanning for signs that people may feel uncomfortable, or need an invitation to contribute, asking people to respond to the observation. When dealing with topics that are potentially distressing, this attentiveness helps to re-establish a balance in the mood of the room and make sure that everyone is leaving with a sense of accomplishment through participation, and possible contacts for support afterward. Enabling participants to deliberate with care (Barnes, 2008; Ward and Barnes, 2015) is part of what is necessary to enabling careful research practice.

I (Tula) applied the integrity of care to understand the different courses of action available to me and the possible outcomes they would have while working on the alcohol and drug service evaluation. A strong pull was to work in solidarity with the Kaupapa Māori (by Māori for Māori) service for young people because the reality was that if that service was removed, there was no other that the community could access in the rural area. As is usual in a service evaluation, adherence to the therapy model was a central concern and came up for discussion where there were demands on practitioners to work in a way that did not fit with their values. One example was where the practitioner working in strict adherence to the approach would be expected to discourage all contact with any family members who were deemed problematic, for example if they had access to drugs. The Māori practitioners talked about sidestepping some aspects of the model that would not be acceptable to *whānau*. The team discussed how to present this as the evaluation was strongly focused on adherence with the model and practitioners were clearly prioritising other values in some cases. Rather than frame it as a lack of adherence, the discussion focused on how the model needed to be adapted to work with Māori.

Research that operates in different cultural contexts requires particular forms of care in the way in which it is conducted. For Ruth, working in different countries in Africa, one of the key issues was the need to explore what the word care itself means in different cultural contexts. She talked about illuminating conversations as the team worked through different understandings of care and what this meant for research investigating caring practices. One project involved a Senegalese researcher with whom it was helpful to understand concepts from different worldviews, and interpretations of concepts in different languages. Ruth provided the example of the concept of child fosterage – translated as *I gave my child to my sister*, for example, a much more informal position than is expected in adoption processes elsewhere. She also noted that in French, care translates as *taking care of* which often means practical support, such as financial support, rather than a focus on caring process and relationality. These conversations among research team members from different sociocultural backgrounds were insightful to affirm the differences and similarities in meanings and thus strengthen the team's capacity to interpret what those they interviewed said to them. As well as linguistic comparisons Ruth also gave the example of the expectation of restraint of emotional reactions in bereavement in Senegal which equated to the British idea of the 'stiff upper lip'. Ruth reflected how the Senegalese researcher was brought onto the project for certain parts of it, but that it would have been better to have them throughout the project for conceptual interpretation during analysis, as well as for language interpretation in the data collection and transcription. She recommended making sure that there is always plenty of time for these discussions throughout research projects. In this project, the team, comprising British, Burkinabe/Belgian and Senegalese researchers, interviewed each other about the death of a relative in their own families and held reflexive conversations about cultural practices surrounding death in preparation for data collection. This influenced the broader cross-cultural approach in the project, including the design of the interview schedules and interpretations of participants' experiences. It allowed discussion of cultural worldviews, the emotionality of the research project and explicit recognition of the research as emotional work. Part of the discussion centred on how personal experiences and recollections have a direct influence on the way a research project is conducted and experienced by the researchers.

Another aspect of process is choosing where to conduct the research. Interviews can be challenging for people with dementia because recall is problematic when memory is affected. I worked on a project in the south of England that employed walking interviews to examine GPS acceptability with people living with memory loss (Bartlett and Brannelly, 2019). The project also had sit-down interviews with the person concerned and family members, if they were available. The difference in walking with the person rather than asking questions in a sit-down interview was remarkable. In the walking interview, the person was more talkative, engaged in the locality, explaining connections, but also talking about themselves, the impact of their condition on them and their concerns about the future. One person asked me every time we met how she seemed and whether I thought she had deteriorated. She showed me her beautiful oil paintings of landscapes and digressed about how people encouraged her to do her art as therapy, which reminded her of her loss as she saw the deterioration in her ability. Another woman pointed out a care home where she visited friends previously and wondered whether she would eventually live there. Two of the men told me that they understood the strain they put on their partners and how they held back from talking about how they felt anxious or worried about their future as it would be upsetting. Despite having worked and researched with people with dementia for many years, this simple shift in setting enabled conversations that I had never been able to previously, and a reciprocal relationship was established that is so often missing when a person is cognitively impaired.

Taking care of the people involved in research was the other concern during our conversations with other researchers and it is to this that we now turn. One of the ways in which this happens is checking in with people, offering space for debriefing and sharing observations and interpretations when collecting the data or at key points in the life of the research project.

## Taking care of the people

When doing research, the ethics of care calls for care for the people involved. In this section we provide some examples of the ways in which care was an explicit aim during research to bring attention to the approaches we think have helped people stay involved, to view that involvement as a worthwhile endeavour, and which were a necessity in enabling new insights and understandings. The research that we draw on is often about an experience of vulnerability such as illness, disability or the need for increased support, including using health and social care services. The people who co-research in this context are likely to experience some challenges and need flexibility and support to stay involved in the work. For others, the research may be emotional work that needs to be acknowledged and cared for throughout the process. The people we spoke to recognise the need for support for all members of the team, including the researchers. Ruth noted that research ethics committees are likely to ask about support for research participants when researching sensitive topics, but that this does not extend to the research team. This is despite the fact that in participatory research there is usually a clear link between personal experience and the research topic. In recent research bids, Ruth had included a budget for counselling or supervision costs for the research team, including community peer researchers, as well as participants. This is to enable support through research funding in recognition of the emotional toll that doing research may take, and to have access to help for team members to work through their personal reactions to the issues that may be raised.

An ethics of care approach ensures attentiveness to people's preferences about how to contribute. This seems obvious, but research projects often run to tight deadlines without enough prior consideration given to how people may like to contribute. To support involvement, it is necessary to know a lot about people's lives and what is going on for them as this will affect how they will be able to join in. It needs ongoing attentiveness through the way introductions are made; the time provided in meetings for people to talk about things other than the task in hand, as well as careful listening and checking in with people between meetings. In the wellbeing project this came to be referred to as 'backstitching'. Bea would meet with Lizzie Ward, the university research fellow, and sometimes also with Marian to review what had happened in meetings; consider whether anyone had appeared unsure or upset and follow up with them if needed; to review whether the process had worked or whether any adjustment in ways of working was necessary. Bunty's reflections of the way in which team members shared phone numbers, and sometimes contacted each other if they were uncertain or wanted to talk through what had happened, indicated that a similar informal process developed among co-researchers as well. We can see all phases of the process of care reflected here. There was an attentiveness to needs of team members resulting in an acceptance of responsibility for competent action with an ongoing awareness of how participants were responding to taking part. This all contributed to the building of solidarity within the team.

One example of a situation where a co-researcher was unable to attend to carry out research tasks was when they phoned from a hospital ward on a day of scheduled research interviews. My (Tula's) previous mental health nursing practice background was helpful here. The co-researcher had been detained under the Mental Health Act for the past few days and was not allowed out of the hospital ward. We discussed why he was detained and what he could do about it. There was a meeting planned for later that day where the hospital team suggested that he move onto a different Section of the Act that he was unfamiliar with, and we talked through the consequences of that. Our discussion enabled some clarity about the implications of the proposed change, and he went to the meeting to ask to be released from the Section which, after review, was granted, and he re-joined the research project. We discussed how he wanted to continue to contribute, and what support might be needed. Having options for the levels of commitment people can offer, and flexibility in how people want to contribute, helps people stay involved, even if their contribution changes.

The different contexts in which research projects happen have possible associated areas of concern that researchers need to look out for. Ceri talked about the team's responsibilities to care for each other through the time that they are together, to be explicit about the need for care within the team which she thought was undervalued. Ceri recognised that researchers in colonial societies need to be alert to the likelihood of the experience of historical or intergenerational trauma because of colonisation, which is something that is becoming more visible in coloniser societies. Researchers need to know how to support people, and this is usually through connections with local indigenous peoples through community organisations. People are at different stages of understanding these historical impacts and being involved in research could be the mechanism by which another layer of understanding is unearthed. Offering some connection to others with similar experiences can be an opportunity for repair. Ceri reflected on the importance of hearing histories and experiences of trauma in a human-to-human connection that breaks down the barriers of the 'researched' versus the researcher. We think it is particularly helpful when the trauma is acknowledged as part of the research in the way that the person who has experienced it agrees with. This implies a capacity and willingness to demonstrate care in difficult circumstances.

I (Marian), Bea and Bunty (together with Lizzie Ward) worked together over a number of projects and years. As one project was completed others were identified and research proposals were co-created. Care within the team was implicit through the relationships developed over time. Bea's role included emotional and practical support for the volunteers at Age UK, and this extended into the research roles they took on during this collaboration. Having a deep understanding of the factors that influenced older people's involvement as volunteers, Bea understood when this was working well and when it was not. Considerable attention was paid to the practical issues of transport to get to meetings and reminders being sent out to check people were still OK to attend. Time is needed for non-research-related discussions, getting to know people, how they are, how the day-to-day of life is going for them. All of the people we spoke to recognised this need. In the introduction to this second part of the book I (Marian) noted how I learnt this in my first major project that adopted participatory methods. Working with people caring for ill or disabled relatives in a research project, it was important to allow space for people to talk about their everyday experiences of caregiving and for team members to offer support to each other in response. Bunty noted the importance of supportive relationships within the research team and that this encompassed both support from Bea, Lizzie and Marian, as well as the support that developed among the co-researchers. Her reference to the importance of starting team meetings with conversation over coffee and cake reflects what Iris Marion Young (2000) describes as the process of 'greeting' in her critique of deliberation as a process solely of rational argumentation and debate. Both Bunty and Liz referred to developing friendships as an important part of being involved. Listening and learning from others requires being prepared to listen to people who may speak in very different ways and this is something that all members of the team may need to learn. As an older person, Bunty relished a slower pace so that the conversation could be followed and to hear about how others think about things, even if people went off at tangents and took some time to tell their story. But this had not suited everyone. Two younger members of the research team, both in their mid-60s, had dropped out before the project was complete, in part because they were frustrated at the slow pace.

As projects progress, more in-depth discussions between the team can help relational care develop. The time spent getting to know each other earlier in the project means that people know who it is they will turn to for help. People accrue synergies and connections, and where people are less experienced, wisdom from others. Ceri gave an example of a young researcher who found it difficult to hear stories from disabled people about the impact of welfare cuts, as she was not aware of the reality of the conditions of life for the people who were affected. Conducting a research interview may be the first time that researchers encounter a person who is homeless, older, living with mental health challenges, or in poverty, for example. Preparation for collecting data in situations which may be confronting or unknown is good practice to anticipate potential situations and enable people to prepare for the work, emotionally and cognitively. Ceri talked about how the young researcher felt uneasy leaving the person in a poor state and was worried for them. This is a familiar response from more experienced as well as newer researchers. Team leaders have a responsibility to listen and respond to researchers in this situation and to come to a mutual agreement about what is possible in order to minimise harms. Ceri reflected that one way to break down boundaries is to have discussions that acknowledge that everyone feels troubled by these experiences and this shared discussion allows less experienced researchers to see the reactions and responses of more experienced researchers. Bunty reflected on her role as a co-researcher over the years she was involved with the university. Bunty had been a counsellor, and one of the aspects of doing research that was uncomfortable for her was not being able to offer more help to the people that she interviewed. Bunty reflected that she continued to find that a real difficulty when looking back on the research – that she knew she had a way of helping but had not been able to offer this in this context. I (Tula) interviewed a couple who were living with dementia, and the relationship was under strain as the husband had stopped talking to his wife. She was very frustrated that he was able to talk to other people but not to her. I discussed this with him during the walking interview and he was encouraged to share his thoughts when we got back to the house. He did so and there was a shift in the tension between them. This was possible because the research involved multiple visits, seven in total over the course of the research, and there was time to spend with them to have these conversations. An ethics of care approach would justify taking care where you can in the research process.

We have more roles in research than as investigators. Among other research relationships are the 'stranger' relationships associated with roles as reviewers. In our conversation with Viv she raised the value of undertaking these roles with care, a reimagining of our responsibilities in a more collaborative and relational way that is less distanced than is currently encouraged. Viv talked about how these roles could be practised differently with ethics of care thinking, having written extensively about achieving socially just pedagogy, rethinking privilege and moving towards embedded reciprocal relationships which we inhabit together (see, for example, Bozalek et al, 2016; Leibowitz and Bozalek, 2016). Academics frequently take a collaborative approach to research and work in inter- or post-disciplinary environments where collaboration is essential. But in the context of reviewing research proposals or journal articles, a more competitive culture often prevails.

This conversation prompted us (Marian and Tula) to consider our experiences of receiving reviews and of reviewing. Our experiences are that peer review practices vary in expectation and practice. As academics we expect critique and welcome suggestions that peers make to strengthen the work. We experience rejection of journal articles and grant applications and, however often this happens and however senior we become, it can still hurt. Responses from reviewers are sometimes overly critical, or indicate that the work has been read through an interpretive lens that we do not share. While there is a strong expectation that we will learn though failure, rejection can not only mean that months of hard work seem to be wasted, but it can also leave us feeling vulnerable and struggling to achieve resilience. We reflected on our own practices as reviewers as academics committed to collaboration and empowerment. We have received guidance that includes advice such as the journal only publishes a small number of submissions so expect to reject articles that are submitted for review, or funding for new projects being limited to 10 per cent of submissions so to look for flaws that can justify rejection. The competition model for funding creates lots of losers and few winners. For one person to be funded there must be many more who are unsuccessful. But many of the projects are worthwhile and fundable. So how we communicate this and the comments and feedback provided on submissions is really important to show care for the person who has taken the time, effort and energy to submit the proposal. Suggestions and encouragement are needed. Reviewing then becomes a task of identifying strength and potential improvements that support the reworking of the submission if it is not quite there yet.

One way of supporting people is to extend the reviewer role out to the academic community prior to submission, through supporting writing in preparation for submission. I (Tula) set up an ethics committee support group as part of a wider mental health research group in Wellington. Health and university ethics committees were so protectionist about access to people with mental health problems, that most research was refused and researchers were discouraged. The support group commented on applications before they were submitted to revise any content we thought would deny access. But we have also experienced 'advice' from university colleagues that has not been helpful: because the person might have a lot of experience of securing research funding, but in very different fields to those we have been working in and has very little context-specific understanding of the kind of issues we have been exploring in this book. A careful approach to reviewing requires relevant competence.

## Conclusion

In our experience of doing ethics of care research and in our conversations with the contributors to this book, there were some really striking examples of what working together on projects means and how people consider their participation. We hope these are helpful examples of the kinds of thinking and action taken to care more through the process of research. Taking care with that process is essential as it has immediate influence on the project but also longer-term consequences for what people take from the experience of being involved in research. Doing research often involves emotion work for ourselves and others we involve in this process. Sometimes the emotions generated are unexpected. They may emerge from our exposure to the unfamiliar and distressing experiences of others, and they may tap into our own forgotten, hidden or unacknowledged personal experiences. In some cases we open up spaces in which others reveal their haunting by systemic or historical oppressions. The overly functional requirements of research ethics committees often do not acknowledge the unpredictable issues that emerge during the process of the work. They do not prepare us sufficiently to care, nor do they provide a framework within which we can develop caring research practices.

We are reflecting as two White women who have done research in different contexts, sometimes with people who have questioned our legitimacy to research beyond our lived experience, often working with people whose objective circumstances render them in a less powerful position in relation to research than we occupy. The ethics of care asks us to be attentive to the particular context in which we seek to enact research as a caring practice, but also to recognise that care receivers contribute to the process and that building solidarity is part of the purpose. How we achieve that will be different if we are working with people using mental health services, with migrant mothers, older people who have a lifetime of professional experience, or family members responding to bereavement in sub-Saharan Africa. We can learn from ways in which different groups have generated ways of doing research that reflect what matters to them: both in terms of substance and method. For example, indigenous research has specific approaches, such as Kaupapa Māori that draws on Te Ao Māori and *tikanga* to enable people to feel at home in the research area, and to counter previous harms from western approaches. In colonised societies it is also necessary to bring awareness to the relationship between the people and the land, to consider the place in which the research happens and the responsibility to reciprocate with the community for that. Creative approaches flatten hierarchies in research teams when all team members are participants in activities together and contribute together. Bringing in others with skills in theatre or poetry provides a spark to the research, and enables researchers to be part of the group with the team. This change in role enables researchers to spend more time in discussion to understand the research from other perspectives in more depth. Democratising research aims to ensure that all voices are heard to steer and shape the research. An ethics of care approach helps unpack and explore embedded and complex situations to find solutions.

# 7

# Analysis, legacy and care

In this chapter, the focus is on doing analysis of data together; some examples of the kinds of legacies that come from being involved in research; the ways in which researchers recognise the needs of the communities in which they are involved and look to reciprocate involvement; and how to end involvement well. We provide examples of approaches to analysis where the people we spoke to discuss how to co-produce analysis, how to present the work to co-researchers to do analysis together, providing space for people to engage with the data and connect the experience of data collection with analysis. Working together on data analysis is enabled by researchers creating accessible formats, techniques and support for people with experience to contribute. We provide examples of the talking points and negotiated outcomes that happen during this process, recognising that room is needed for disagreements, that research is producing new knowledge that might not be palatable to everyone. Collaboration to complete a project includes interpreting data together, prioritising findings, report and publication production, and collaborative dissemination events and practices. Co-researchers may have had experience to draw on that relate to these activities in previous professional roles, such as public speaking, report writing or other creative skills such as poetry, theatre or visual arts. They may also be involved in campaigning and policy influencing and so have access to people and spaces that will help communicate findings to those who need to know. We revisit the value of care – to pay attention, listen carefully and respond to find an acceptable way forward. We discuss examples where the ethics of care was not the explicit framework for the research, but has been used as a reflective tool when it comes to analysis. An explicit ethics of care analytic process, Selma Sevenhuijsen's helpful 'Trace' (2003) is discussed as an example of a systematic care ethics approach to the analysis of policy or text documents that seeks out the philosophical underpinnings and the implicit and explicit assumptions about care that they contain.

Part of the work of analysis and dissemination is being able to describe, interpret and translate experiences of one group to tell another audience what that is like. This has its challenges. I (Marian) recounted an experience when starting out on a book about the Pilsdon Community where I am currently volunteering and became involved in an oral history to mark its 60th anniversary (Barnes et al, 2022). The community offers a safe space for people with addictions and mental health problems and is grounded in the Christian faith of its members (a faith I do not share). One of the, very thoughtful, trustees expressed some concern that writing about it would somehow undermine what is most important about the community. Another member of the community used the word 'ineffable' to suggest that it was not possible to describe it, concerned that by seeking to 'capture' the community in writing, what is special about it becomes lost. Associated with this was a concern that through documenting everyday lives of those who have been part of the community, it somehow becomes fixed at the level of what is observable and this is not helpful. To counter this, in the book we say, in a number of different ways, that the community is constantly being made and that the book is part of the process of storying and re-storying a living place. It is one of many different narratives that both sustain and develop a place that is constantly changing, yet remains true to its core values. In writing about it we attempt to make the 'ineffable effable'. For social scientists, a key aspect of the work we do is to understand and communicate different lives, different ways of feeling, thinking, different values and experiences, and what they mean for how we live together. It is often hard to do but we search for different ways of doing it. And as one of the current members of the Pilsdon Community observed about the way in which I and my co-authors were writing the book, if we do this with love, then our different starting points and different beliefs are not problematic. This observation reflects the criterion of indigenous peoples that research should show love for future generations.

We have argued that the way impact is defined and measured is driven by the needs of the university and broader scientific community, rather than by the people who are affected by research. Here, we discuss legacies as a way of capturing the influences and implications of being involved in research, both for the individuals involved but also across time and projects. We suggest that an ethics of care calls for recognition of knowledge as treasure that is located with the people who hold it and valuable to the communities it resides with. Part of the legacy that research leaves behind is the reciprocity that researchers offer communities; what people give back to the communities that have contributed to the projects that can support the communities' aims. Finally in this chapter, the focus is on endings of relationships between the people affected by the research project, and making sure that the communities that have been involved are informed about research findings and the possibilities for change that come from them.

## Doing analysis with an ethics of care

Doing analysis that includes multiple perspectives needs to be planned and organised to decide how best to incorporate those perspectives. We (Tula and Marian) have both done qualitative or mixed method projects with co-researchers whose involvement included co-analysis of data. Others that we spoke to for this book have done participatory qualitative work that has included analysis or discussion of findings. The contributions of co-researchers to the initial framing of projects and to detailed design of data collection in ways that will be sympathetic to people with whom they share experiences can be extended to the process of analysis. But many will be unfamiliar with working with data in this way and so care needs to be taken in planning and supporting this process. Not everyone will be comfortable with working with data and some may want to comment on findings rather than work through the data themselves. Ethics of care thinking opens the space for people to contribute in the way that they want, and relational care at this stage of the process will facilitate the inclusion of multiple perspectives as the team discuss meanings and interpretations. Throughout the project people will have become entangled in the data. This is the point at which threads are drawn together to create a pattern that is created from the different contributions made to the project. Here, we give examples of different ways in which people have been involved in the analysis of data and prioritising findings from the research.

We start with my (Marian's) reflection on setting the scene to create the right ambiance where people feel comfortable and able to contribute to analysis. This needs to recognise that this may well be an activity that is new to people and, while they may find this stimulating, it may also generate anxiety. Working together over a period of months or years builds a sense of collective responsibility for the delivery of good quality research. This is achieved by making sure everyone is supported to participate as fully as they want to, but not asked to take on tasks they do not feel happy with. The research group carrying out the project on older people and wellbeing developed new skills and tried new research techniques which built confidence over time. Some of the co-researchers were involved in the process of analysing the rich data from interviews and focus groups, but not everyone wanted to take on the detailed task of analysis. We looked for ways in which all could contribute without making demands that some did not feel comfortable with. There was an initial open discussion in team meetings about the topics that had been discussed in the interviews undertaken by the co-researchers. Based on this identification of key topics, the research fellow, Lizzie Ward, coded transcripts and sorted material into documents based on thematic codes. Some members of the team then took these documents in order to look at themes relevant to their interests. At later team meetings the co-researchers then presented their reflections and interpretations of the material they had been looking at and these were explored further in discussions involving the whole team. These discussions enabled emotional responses to some of the issues interviewees had spoken about to be expressed, as well as a space in which team members could talk about some of their own experiences that they had been reminded of by the data. This iterative process thus involved people in different ways to generate deep insights into what mattered to people. The significance of care to wellbeing was evident both from the interview content and the responses this evoked. Collating and writing up the themes in a research report was done primarily by Lizzie and Marian. This was followed by journal articles and a book in which the ethics of care was applied to enable a further level of interpretative analysis of both interview content and research process (Barnes et al, 2018). Alongside the writing of the research report, there was a concurrent process where a lay version of the findings was created. In this separate process, some team members worked with Bea to produce a document called 'As Time Goes By'. This was intended as a research output that was written by old people for old people with the aim of sharing experiences of how to sustain wellbeing in old age. Its design and format reflected its different purpose and it was distributed directly to old people via the voluntary organisation's networks. It was a practical expression of solidarity between the research team and others they might not know, but who they wanted to benefit from the research.

The researchers we spoke to talked about different ways in which they prepared data to engage discussion with co-researchers, participants or advisory groups, identifying careful thinking about facilitating ideas and contributions. Umut described a constant gathering of perspectives and ideas throughout the research process, such as the presentation of analysed data at workshops for reflections and observations. Short videos were used to explain the findings, with invitations to people to respond about how they felt about these. There were important insights coming from these workshops, including the rejection of the term migrant, which we discussed in Chapter 6. Similar approaches were described in other projects.

There were also examples of phased analysis to enable people to contribute. In the GPS acceptability study with people with dementia, I (Tula) was part of an interdisciplinary team who analysed interview data to produce the draft findings and discussion. To facilitate analysis of people with experience, some of the participants and the advisory group of people with dementia and family carers were invited to discuss the findings and to help the research team prioritise the key messages from the research. As the project was about walking and being outdoors, the setting was a two-day residential stay in the New Forest with guided walking. The findings were visually presented by an artist and explained to small groups to invite insights and feedback about the project. The key message that the people with dementia advocated strongly for was only using GPS if consent was explicitly given, which would require early introduction of the technology. This informed the reporting and dissemination of the research. A film of the residential stay was created to capture the perspectives of everyone involved about the process of being part of the research. Films, blogs and additional reports are increasingly used to capture and disseminate something of the experience of being involved in research projects.

Being attentive to people means that there is a responsibility to act accordingly in ethics of care thinking. To facilitate analysis in the alcohol and drug service evaluation, I (Tula) organised a two-day meeting to work through the data together as a team. The data was laid out as text excerpts on large sheets of paper so that it could be perused and discussed. As the research team themed the data, all of the data that did not fall into those themes was discussed to make sure we were not excluding anything that the co-researchers thought important. We worked through theme by theme, and the team were asked to connect their experience to the data and provide an idea or interpretation where the data resounded with them. This approach identified a significant difference of interpretation within the team, with extensive talking points. The research overall took a citizenship and care approach, and there was one element of the service provision that the researchers were critical about but that the young people with experience welcomed. In the service, young people are excluded from discussions and decisions that are made about them. It is an intentional approach that takes control from the young person. It included that the young person is not necessarily called on to talk to members of the family or community about what they have been doing (most were in trouble with the police for damage to property or similar). The young people stayed at home with a curfew, and were not allowed to leave the house by their parent or guardian. The researchers favoured an approach that included the perspectives of the young person, that asked them what was troubling them, what they thought about what had happened and helped them to understand their responsibility to themselves and others. But the co-researchers were measuring those actions against different criteria altogether, as they saw being able to stay at home as preferable to being moved into a psychiatric ward or residential placement, possibly forced to do so, as had been the experience they were familiar with. Unequivocally, the young people preferred the sanctions that parents put in place rather than going to a mental health service at the age of 12–16. While the researchers considered participation in the community, the young people saw total exclusion from the community by being moved out of it as the issue. What mattered most to the co-researchers was different to what mattered to the researchers, and a significant learning moment in the project.

This project also raised an important issue of the responsibilities felt by researchers. We needed to be careful in the feedback to the evaluation funders and in the way we framed any critique of the service. It was clear that the services should continue given the lack of resource or alternative available for the families who benefited from the help. The Kaupapa Māori service in particular was supporting people with high levels of need in dire poverty. The need for the service was significant and the families who spoke to the evaluation team were clear that this was a lifeline. The workers in the Kaupapa service helped the families beyond the service, for example through community support at the *marae* to help with food parcels. It was hard to argue with the need for this when visiting families that had no electricity, a lot of mouths to feed and were very grateful for a food package as a thank you for contributing to the evaluation. Reporting back it was clear that there needed to be a very clear statement about the conditions of life that the people who accessed the service were experiencing and the experience of the service as essential support for them. The discussion resulted in a report that emphasised the support received by the families and an article that critiqued the approach for its inclusion of the young people and fit with Te Ao Māori (worldview) (Brannelly et al, 2013b). These examples identify what happened in response to the different perspectives and knowledge in the project. Attentiveness to these perspectives and an acceptance of responsibility to find solutions that responded well to those different positions embodied the commitment of care ethics to not only critique but to renew caring policies and practices.

Tula used the ethics of care as a framework to analyse observed practice and interviews with social workers and community psychiatric nurses in her study of decision making for people with dementia moving to residential care (Brannelly, 2006). The phases of care were used to consider how people with dementia were included in decision making by the practitioners. This included how the practitioners were attentive to needs, facilitated people to be involved, responded to that need and planned care, and how the reaction of people with dementia was instrumental in decisions. Using the ethics of care in this way disrupted one fundamental expectation in the way that practitioners work. It is expected that practitioners include people on the basis of their ability to be included; people are offered participation and if they are unable to contribute then alternative avenues are sought. However, using attentiveness to explore practitioner approaches, it was apparent that some practitioners never offered participation because they believed the person was incapable based on the diagnosis rather than the person's ability, pathologising the person and excluding them from the opportunity to offer a perspective. This was consistent with approaches that objectify the person as socially dead (Brannelly, 2011) and challenged a fundamental understanding of the ethical approaches of practitioners.

Secondary data analysis can also be carried out using the ethics of care as a framework. Charlotte Clarke and colleagues (Clarke et al, 2018b) examined the value of using the ethics of care in participatory analysis of a secondary dataset. The dataset was from a pan-national evaluation of carer and peer support initiatives and the ethics of care guided discussions regarding interpersonal relationships between people with dementia and those who care for them. An alternative lens of risk was also used to interpret the data. The ethics of care-led exploration was framed using the questions (Clarke et al, 2018b, p 1157): How do accounts of interactions between people with dementia, carers and other significant people portray attentiveness, responsibility, competence, responsiveness and trust? What are the interpersonal and societal dynamics described which promote a positive cycle of the ethic of care towards an empowering relationship; or that produce a negative cycle of a disempowering relationship? The ethics of care approach identified that a collaborative, inclusionary approach was useful in overcoming the exclusions that people with dementia face on a daily basis, drawing out an understanding of solidarity that helps people to relax knowing that others are watching out for them, which in turn helps people to be themselves and less fearful of social awkwardness. An accompanying video identifies the analysis of the experience of living with dementia in the community (https://vimeo.com/channels/1148563). Clarke et al's (2018a) use of the ethics of care to draw out and discuss relational care as a means of inclusion for people for dementia and the meanings they attach to it is a novel way of understanding more about the experience of living with dementia, about which relatively little is known given its ubiquity. It is a welcome addition to the ways in which the ethics of care can be used in applied research. Another example within the same field is a study I (Marian) carried out with colleagues evaluating an information and support programme for carers of people with dementia (Barnes and Henwood, 2015). Adopting a care ethics perspective enabled us to interrogate naïve assumptions that better information will automatically lead to better care. Flis Henwood and I argued the necessity to 'inform with care', recognising that the process of receiving and processing information can be personally unsettling and can impact relationships between care givers and care receivers. I have also revisited earlier work on deliberative democracy and social movement action, applying the phases of care analysis to the process of deliberation and exploring the constraining consequences of attempts to distance 'caring about' an issue from deliberative processes (Barnes, 2008, 2019b). In each of these cases care ethics invites us to ask different questions of research data and thus to offer different insights.

As these latter examples suggest, research that was not designed from within an ethics of care perspective can use this in making sense of the material that is generated. In the introduction to this chapter we referred to an oral history project in which I (Marian) became involved in the course of my work as a volunteer in a residential community (Barnes et al, 2022). Oral history uses free form interviews to generate different stories that weave together to create an account of, in this case, a 60-year period during which people with mental health difficulties have lived alongside others in a place where they can seek to repair broken lives. People spoke of what living in community had meant to them, of both the challenges and joys of living and working alongside others, and of the significance of the physical place in which they were living and the animals and plants who shared this with them. The community is explicitly not a provider of care services. But the nature of the relationships formed within this place are key to understanding why it has worked for many who have spent time there and why it has survived for much longer than many other 'alternative' ways of living. Care is integral to the way life is lived in this community: care for other people, for the animals, the soil and the plants that are grown there and that are the source of much of the community's food. And, as one of those who has spent time in the community on and off for many years said, care for the community itself. Reading interview transcripts from within an ethic of care frame offered ways of reflecting on the relational significance of life within the community and the importance of a temporal perspective on care, but also prompted reflection on the limitations of a care perspective that always starts from individuals rather than a collective. In a very different cultural context from that of the Māori about whom Tula writes in this book, the Pilsdon Community also asks us to start from what is necessary to sustain and care for a community so that people can live together as well as possible within it. A care ethics perspective that emphasises the contextual nature of care as a diverse activity can both enhance and enlarge our understanding of care as an ethical, political, personal and interspecies activity necessary to sustaining relational life.

## Trace analysis

Interview transcripts are one type of textual document that we can subject to analysis from an ethic of care. There are others. Care ethics has been used as a critical and transformative perspective from which to view a wide range of policies, including: child and family policies; long-term care for old people; public health; education; international development and many more. Policy analysis is central plank of academic social and public policy and a range of post-positivist approaches have developed that link social theory, politics and sometimes psychosocial analysis (for example Hajer and Wagenaar, 2003; Hunter, 2015). What is distinctive about using the ethics of care as a reference point for the analysis of policy is that this is an explicitly evaluative approach that places care at the centre and interrogates the way in which policies enable or frustrate caring relations. Selma Sevenhuijsen (2003) has also argued that this enables a creativity and capacity to articulate new ways of thinking and activity – that it is transformative.

Sevenhuijsen (2003) developed 'Trace: A method for normative policy analysis from an ethic of care' as a result of undertaking a number of analyses of public health and welfare policies. The method came out of the practice of researching policy rather than preceding it. Focusing on different types of texts that include formal policy documents, organisational mission statements, texts of public policy debates, legal documents and others, she describes the aim as to:

> [T]race the normative framework(s) in policy reports in order to evaluate and renew these from the perspective of an ethic of care. The background motivation to this approach is the wish to further develop care into a political concept and to position care as a social and moral practice in notions of citizenship. (Sevenhuijsen, 2003, p 1)

The full process involves four stages:

1. Establish normative frameworks within the text: based on who produced the text; how the problem is being defined; what are the leading values evident within it; how is human nature understood; if care is explicitly mentioned, how is it defined; the extent to which gender in care is acknowledged; what is the role of the state vis-à-vis private individuals, and what are the rhetorical characteristics of the text.
2. Evaluating: it is inevitable that this will have already been prompted in stage 1 but Sevenhuijsen suggests holding back as much as possible in order to establish a 'fair' judgement. This second stage opens up questions about the political philosophy guiding the text; the adequacy of the way in which the problem is defined, and then an explicit focus on the way in which power and inequality and the way they intersect are addressed.
3. Stage 3 marks what Sevenhuijsen names as the more creative and imaginative step of the process: renewing. How would Fisher and Tronto's definition of caring make a difference to the way this policy is set out? What forms of knowledge is the policy based on? And how would other key aspects of care thinking make a difference? For example, if we understand human life as being characterised by interdependence, vulnerability, the inter-relationship between mind and body, and values that are integral to everyday life, how might we want to renew this policy?
4. The final step involves making concrete the preceding analysis by suggesting specific policy measures.

This very detailed process has implicitly or explicitly guided researchers whose focus has been on a wide range of policy issues. Fiona Williams' work over many years has reflected a similar way of thinking about social policies (2001, 2004, 2021), and in her more recent work identifies care as essential to the response to the multiple challenges facing welfare states. I (Marian) used a rather compressed version in an analysis of UK social care personalisation policies (Barnes, 2011). In principle we could see this as an analysis process that could be undertaken with others who are directly impacted by the policy issues involved. While there is not an inevitable relationship between the aim of constructive renewal and policy change, the process that Sevenhuijsen sets out does demonstrate a real concern that the ethics of care should not be solely a critical way of thinking, or indeed a method, but a *practice*, a way of doing.

## Legacies from research participation

Research is often motivated by the need to improve the conditions of life. Doing ethics of care research intentionally exposes those conditions to find solutions. Attentiveness to the need identifies a responsibility to find a solution, or to draw on Collins (2015), interdependent relationships generate responsibilities. This is particularly the case in research undertaken collaboratively with those impacted by the issues being studied. Researchers may view achieving social change as a long-term outcome as research evidence builds, discourses evolve, policy shifts and practice changes at its often glacial pace. In the social sciences the aim of transformation is commonly cited; in other disciplines the aspiration for social change may be less explicitly stated, such as in health or education research (Rodriguez and Morrison, 2019), but is becoming more usual.

The question of what impact research was having was central to the research programme 'Connected Communities', supported by UK Research Councils. In an edited collection addressing just this issue, Facer and Pahl (2017) noted that, in comparison with attention to making university/community engagements happen, '[m]uch less attention has been paid to understanding the legacy of these moments of collaboration between academics and communities or to how and whether these processes deliver on the significant claims about quality, democracy and equity that such projects are often bound up with' (p 1). The concept of 'legacy' rather than 'impact' was promoted by researchers in this programme as a way of both expanding our understanding of what processes of change actually involve, and of how the value of collaborations can be narrated to sceptical audiences.

Our conversations as authors and with others for this book identified numerous examples of legacies from research involvement. People involved as co-researchers have matured their research and knowledge skills, building research capacity (Neal et al, 2015) as they have been involved in different projects and have contributed both to better understanding of effective practices of involvement, and to building research knowledge. They have also been part of work that has been designed specifically to generate legacies. A second phase of the wellbeing research project that I, Marian, Bea, Bunty and Liz were involved in, continued through Economic and Social Research Council follow-on funding to produce learning resources for social care practitioners based on research findings. This time-limited funding source created a different context in which to work, but enabled a much more developed process of involvement in generating resources to create a lasting legacy from the project. In addition to the old people who had been members of the research team throughout, the group was joined by social care practitioners and this, too, created a different dynamic. And since the decision was to create filmed resources the other person who effectively became a member of the team was a film director. A discussion of this process is included in chapter 8 of Barnes et al (2018). This also offers an in-depth analysis from the perspective of deliberation and the ethics of care. We concluded this discussion by writing:

> [O]ur experience shows that the application of care ethics to collaborations between older people, researchers, and service providers, can enable transformative dialogue about care and its importance to older people, and help ethical awareness and sensibilities amongst practitioners. To realize these aspirations requires understanding such collaborations as involving moral deliberation as well as an exchange of knowledge. ... Taking part can offer old people as well as younger researchers and practitioners an experience of what relational wellbeing consists of and can provide a location in which solidarity can be generated through 'caring with' others (Tronto, 2013). (Barnes et al, 2018, p 170)

Working with Marian and the team, Bea considered the impact that the role had on her personally in terms of developing her knowledge and experience of research. After being involved with these participatory projects, Bea worked with a young medic in training to be a General Practitioner in another project that examined older peoples' lived experience of medication issues. She was able to offer a helpful person-centred perspective that applied ethics of care thinking to the experiences of both older people and of clinicians. The older people identified difficulties with opening medication packaging and reading the information sheets so had trouble taking the medications and knowing what they were for. They also experienced difficulties in being heard in terms of their experiences of the effects of their medication and concerns they had about them. Bea realised there was also limited review of medications which left people with the risks associated with polypharmacy. The ethics of care work provided a way of talking about values and offered a similar way of expressing doubts and anxieties to both older people and frontline staff. Bea described her knowledge of care ethics as translatable into other projects and talked of how it allowed her to make sense of and explain what was important in a way that connected with others' experiences.

The young medic leading the research was doing his PhD and training to specialise in working with older people. He wanted to represent the voices of older people in the research. At the end of the project, Bea was invited to present at the medical school, and opened the event with a focus on the lived experience of clinicians torn by the pressures of time, a common ethical dilemma for medics working with older people (Alzheimer Europe Report, 2015). Bea presented these challenges using the ethics of care to highlight how the context of time pressures did not support good practice, and asking the clinicians to consider their own experiences. She described the feeling of breaking an enormous taboo in the way she reflected on the experiences of care givers (doctors) who could experience a lack of care for themselves in their working lives. Bea was able to draw on the range of research in which she had been involved and that had used care ethics in order to highlight the necessity and complexity of care. She spoke about the way in which people try to be well when they are not well; that people try to provide care when conditions are not supportive of this, and that all of the people involved in caregiving need also to receive care. This was well received by an audience that was unused to such an input. To borrow again from Māori, this is *taonga* (treasure) as Bea has situated, rich, deep knowledge from a multiplicity of sources that influences change and can be clearly seen as a legacy of researching with care.

Umut recounted an example of woman who had been part of the migrant mothers project who later joined a school board and said that being involved in the research had given her the courage to do so. Umut thought it an overstatement to take the credit for that happening, but that the decision was influenced by many factors, including involvement in the project. We (Tula and Marian) have seen co-researchers go on to further study and research roles working in universities in collaboration with academics. As Umut pointed out, the intention is to acknowledge that involvement in research projects may springboard to other activities and this may be viewed as part of the legacy of projects over a longer term. We suggest that this is another example of treasure that stories of research can recount.

We have written about the development of competence through careful work together in the course of carrying out research. In ethics of care thinking, competence also refers to having the resources available to give the care that is needed. In the GPS project building on the involvement of people with dementia, part of the dissemination strategy was to present the research to a parliamentary special committee at Westminster. To enable the person with dementia, Philippa, to discuss the topic, a question-and-answer session was facilitated by her supporter, Elizabeth. Philippa eloquently and passionately told the committee that no one with dementia should be tracked without their consent, and that facilitating consent required early intervention to offer people with dementia all sorts of community supports that would allow them to stay at home. The resources needed to support the group to attend the parliamentary meeting, and for the overnight stay to take part in the analysis process, were a considerable proportion of the research budget. In research as in other caring contexts a practical commitment from funders is also necessary. Philippa and others went on to contribute to a book about living at home with dementia through interviews about issues that affected them, such as gene testing for hereditary forms of dementia and dealing with the anxiety of memory loss (Bartlett and Brannelly, 2018). Many of the advisory group adopted carrying a GPS so they could be found if they got lost out walking alone. Another legacy of the project was learning from the way the research was carried out. Assessments for the suitability of using GPS have changed to walking with the person, rather than a sit-down interview at home. In a further public engagement activity with the group, I (Tula), artist Cathy Garner and two PhD students, Amelia Abbott and Phillipa Collins, visited people with dementia and their family at home to talk about their lives and create biographical portraits. The aim was to destigmatise the fear that some young people can have of talking to people with dementia, and to show how it is normalised within the lives of people who experience it. The conversations were filmed on a laptop, and edited into a short film, a low-tech DIY approach (www.yout ube.com/watch?v=7G3U6yrlU-Q&t=6s). Copies of the portraits were given to the participants, and these were proudly hung in living rooms and even used at funerals. The emphasis was to show care in the lives of the people, and that this was the most important concern for them, appreciated by the families and the researchers.

For university researchers their teaching is an important space in which their research can create a legacy. Viv led a faculty-wide care ethics course which was an introduction to the philosophy of care for all first-year health and social care students. Some students appreciated Selma Sevenhuijsen's work on care ethics, while others struggled to see its relevance. The course considered issues such as infant mortality from a multidisciplinary perspective and enabled students to think through justice from both care ethics and principle ethics perspectives. Ruth talked about how a small student placement project commissioned by the local council about experiences of loneliness and social isolation among a range of vulnerable groups was influential as the recommendations were adopted by the local council. From a university perspective, the small, local student project was not viewed as proper or rigorous research and holds very little status despite having the ability to realise real-world change.

As we have argued in earlier chapters, our interdependent relational care with others through research comes from a place of personal, intellectual and political connection. We and the people we work with are changed through the processes of being together and learning from each other. But we also need to accept that our responsibilities include an intentional reciprocity with community groups who generously contribute to research. An ethics of care approach values responses that help marginalised communities and there were examples of this in our conversations. Beyond the research projects, relationships are sustained through giving back to communities. Ruth is active with local refugee and minority ethnic organisations, contributing to setting up the university's partnership with the City of Sanctuary and involvement through governance. Umut recognised that the groups she worked with were living in such precarity that focus must be in the day to day rather than future aspirations. In this context reciprocity needs to focus on immediate needs rather than future change. Marian and Bea's partnership supported Bea in steering her hesitant organisation in the direction of identifying those groups who were not on the radar of policy makers and therefore marginalised. Bea acknowledged how tiring and physically demanding it can be to advocate for people. But being in an ongoing relationship of care in these research projects helped sustain her in seeking the change that is needed.

Viv discussed how a relational ontology means it is impossible to separate self from the communities with whom you engage (Bozalek and Zembylas, 2017). The issue of 'identity' has become an increasingly fraught one in political discourse. For many of those we have worked with as researchers, research has been one space in which to assert a positive identity from what has previously been a marginalised or stigmatised position. I (Marian) encountered this in what were sometimes quite uncomfortable ways through early work with disability activists. This included being told that any discussions about gender, 'race' or sexuality in the context of disability activism were disallowed because the priority was to promote shared experiences of disability. This was before I had encountered ideas of intersectionality and I struggled to work out how to respond to this silencing. I have also experienced having my authority to research disability and survivor activism questioned because I do not identify as disabled. Having 'found' feminist care ethics, this helped me in both understanding some of the issues at stake in these challenges, and working out where I stood in relation to them. The ethical, political and theoretical insights have enabled me to reflect on the often ambiguous and complex issues that impact on us as researchers when we enter worlds that we care about, but in which we are outsiders – at least at the time. Our relationships to those issues we research may well change: we grow older, we may become ill or disabled, we may both give and receive care. How we respond to our changing circumstances can be one legacy of the research we do, but this is rarely something that is reflected in impact studies.

## Good endings

Bea brought our attention to the need for good endings to research relationships. Projects end but relationships often endure. Co-researchers and researchers may have lengthy connections to each other through multiple research projects, creating new projects and applying for funding alongside or between projects. Researchers may continue to be in touch with co-researchers and advisers with updates from the research project, to share and celebrate publications. Situations may arise during projects where team members are unable to continue but stay in contact with the group as friends and supporters of each other. We need to be attentive to the way people respond to both planned and unplanned endings, and whether people want to be involved in the future. People leaving the team can mean reconfiguring responsibilities within the group. Marian and Bea reflected on how some members of the team did not stay with the research and how those who continued with the project accepted and shared responsibilities in a way that generated solidarity. Experience of endings can be unpredictable. Although researchers may think they have explained the parameters of the project and when it will end, this may still be felt as a loss by people who have found solidarity in being part of the group. Marian reflected on working with two groups of carers on an early project and having said from the start that this was a time-limited endeavour. A year after the project had ended she met one of the people involved who said she had felt abandoned when it ended. Having taken care of people during the project, an abrupt ending may be experienced as a lack of care, and gentler endings may be needed. And it can be hard to show care in some circumstances, such as when the contact a researcher has with a group of prospective co-researchers is to present a funding proposal for discussion, and then return to give the news that the project was not funded.

Care ethics can inform how to accommodate endings and continuings by attentiveness to the group and what they want to do. The context in which we carry out research impacts the relationships we have with others while we do the work, and the possibilities to leave a positive legacy. As we reflected on what an ethics of care perspective means when applied to research, I (Marian) had been thinking a lot about different ways in which being entangled with people and topics impacts the issues we have been exploring here. My early research projects were undertaken as an employee of service-providing organisations, with the expectation that the research would directly inform policy and service development. This meant my research was embedded in specific organisational and policy contexts and the way in which the research was framed reflected this. It was only later, when I was working in an academic environment, that more theoretical factors became prominent and, while there was greater freedom to define research topics, the connection between findings and outcomes became more tenuous. I developed as a researcher with the assumption and expectation that research would be quite closely linked to change, albeit within a limited environment. In my first project as a university research fellow, I was employed to undertake an evaluation study of an innovative community care project. Although employed by a university I was embedded in the local authority, had a physical base there and worked closely with council and health service employees involved in the project. Thus, for example, a woman employed in the council worked with me on the carers' project discussed and this enabled support for carers' groups to continue beyond the timescale of the research. Working closely with these carers and with other service user groups also meant becoming entangled with those who were critical of the extent to which the project was achieving significant change. Such entanglements are not without problems. The director of the overall project, who went on to develop a significant national profile, was not happy with critiques emerging from the evaluation as she was entirely committed to the underlying values of the project. But it was only through being attentive to different voices during the course of the project that it became possible to pose questions that reflected what mattered to different project participants. Recognising that people care about things in different ways and from different positions is one of the things that the relational ontology of care ethics can help us think through. When we are in the middle of a project and negotiating the relational dynamics as well as the technical challenges of research it can be hard to work out the best or right thing to do. The ethics of care can provide a helpful framework and language within which we can have those conversations that are necessary to demonstrate that we care even if we disagree.

## Conclusion

We hope that sharing our own reflections and those of others has offered real-life insights into what researching with care involves throughout the process. We are pleased to be able to include Bea, Bunty and Marian's reflections on working together to explicate three perspectives on this experience, and recognise the limitations of not being able to reflect multiple perspectives in other cases.

Both of us have used the ethics of care as an analytic tool in research, to examine with people what is and what is not care, and to understand its significance to both wellbeing and social justice. It invites us to ask different questions and to be more aware of the importance of relational factors rather than solely individual concerns. We see the value in the 'Trace' method for assessing how different philosophical positions are represented in policy texts and have undertaken critical policy analysis with the aim of both evaluating and renewing policy. We share a commitment to careful research that leaves a positive legacy for those involved both directly and indirectly.

We especially call for attentiveness to the ways in which people want to participate, working to strengths and offering opportunities for development. Doing the work together, developing knowledge, and building and sustaining capability is a form of *taonga* (treasure) that highlights the importance of reciprocal rather than exploitative relationships in research. Bringing attention to the end of research projects is important to mark the relational care involved, but also to make sure that it is well planned and a part of the process that is not overlooked as we rush on to the next thing. In the final chapter, we reflect further on aspects of the ethics of care and research that have been particularly influential to our thinking, and draw attention to what we think is essential for ethics of care research.

# Reflections on researching with care

In this final chapter, we each personally reflect on how the ethics of care has influenced our thinking about research over our research careers. We also horizon-scan for what we think are important considerations for future ethics of care research. Throughout this book, we have drawn on the work of Gilligan (1982) to ask whose voice is present in research and to consider how the story of research is told; and we have drawn on the work of Tronto (1993, 2013) to argue for recognition of interdependencies in research and of experience as essential knowledge. Our argument is that a critical understanding of the role of care in the world means that we need to not only research the place and meaning of care in diverse contexts and situations, but that we also need to practice research with care. We research the things we care about as moral beings: it is a practice that is personal, political and intellectual. We argue for critical engagement that examines whose voice is heard in decisions about what is researched, in what way and what actions flow from this. We recognise what we have learnt from researching with users of mental health services, old people, family carers and others too often categorised as subjects of research. And we take encouragement from the work of indigenous scholars such as Linda Tuhiwai Smith (1999/2012) who has clearly stated the limitations of research that does not engage in the knowledge frameworks of indigenous people. Research has a responsibility to aid efforts of decolonisation, not add to them and to repair harms rather than reinforce experiences of being subjected to investigation. How research is framed has been a constant concern. We need to become better at avoiding deficit-based framing that is offensive to the people involved and to those they care about, and to work sensitively with the people with whom we engage in research.

Our purpose is not to propose a blueprint, but based on our own experiences and those shared with us by the people we spoke to for Part II of this book, we suggest it is helpful to ask key questions about how to approach the research you are about to do and what to do when unexpected situations arise. These are not methodological questions, but rather invite thoughtfulness about research as a relational practice that can facilitate repair and transformation. The questions we suggest are helpful are shown in Box 8.1.

We provide the example questions in Box 8.1 so that you may be able to orientate research practices by thinking with care ethics to plan and review the approaches, framing and thinking you bring to research. They do not

---

### Box 8.1:  Questions to guide researching with care

- What do you care about and why do you care about it?
- How do you decide what to research and why?
- Why does it matter to you? Was it something that you had personal experience of?
- Why do you want to carry out this project or get involved in it when invited to do so?
- How do you define the topic/questions and who is involved in that?
- What was the process of getting from initial idea to detailed questions and design?
- To what extent did your ideas develop during this phase and what/who contributed to that?
- What did you want to achieve by doing this research? What do others want to achieve by being involved?
- How will you host and be hospitable during the project?
- How will you know that the people in the research are cared for?
- Why might people need care and at what junctures in the research?
- How might you capture the legacies that the research precipitates?
- What outcomes do the people involved in the research want from the research and how might these influence action towards the end of, and beyond, the research?
- What can you offer as reciprocity for the involvement given by those who get involved in the research?

In addition, Smith (1999/2012, pp 175–176) asks:

- To whom is the research accountable?
- For whom is the study worthy and relevant? Who says so?
- What knowledge will the community gain from the study?

---

presume any particular research method, nor any particular context for a project. You will want to think about particular aspects of the research context and the relationships they imply that will suggest more specific questions. For example, how different languages used by members of the research team and others might require care over interpretation and understanding, or how attentiveness to ways in which exposure to difficult life experiences may be necessary to understand how people respond to taking part – as researchers or research participants. Applying the phases of care and the values associated with these to the research process offers a framework and a language in which to reflect throughout the course of any project.

We are grateful to Linda Tuhiwai Smith for allowing us to include her research poem (www.youtube.com/watch?v=dxoJse2a9NE). We have included it here in its entirety as it says so much about the repercussions of poor research practices on indigenous people. Where there is poor framing of research, laden with assumptions of deficit and discrimination, poor research will follow. This poem relates specifically to the context of colonisation. As we explored in Chapter 2 the precise dynamics of relationships between knowledge and justice vary, but all involve the interplay between power, domination and the capacity to determine valid knowledge. Smith captures this from her perspective as an indigenous woman, but also connects with other struggles in which research has been implicated in causing rather than repairing harms. We offer it as a reminder to researchers in all contexts.

*Research Ethics for Indigenous People 101* by Linda Tuhiwai Smith

It began long before
the Holocaust's scientists
experimented on Jews, Gypsies
and others they hated,
Before their industrial scale genocide
Brought modernity down
And Nuremberg set out a Code
It began long before
Tuskegee
The deliberate infecting of Syphilis
Into black men's bodies
To study their 'Bad Blood'
Science voyeurs
Watching the method at work
killing their participants
one
by one
by one
It began long before
the Havasupai
had their DNA taken under one guise
And used against them under another
Taking from the sick to feed the well
Simply because they believed their moral right to do so
It began long before
the Portuguese had improved their instruments of navigation
enabling them to sail beyond their imaginations
It began
Before Columbus left Spain's harbours
Before Cook set sail for Tahiti
Before slave traders and missionaries crossed the Atlantic and
the Pacific

Before the great synergy of capitalism, science, nation building
and empire
Before the Doctrine of Discovery legitimated and
fuelled Europe's
Quest for eternity
It began long before the slaughter, enslavement,
And genocide of Native Peoples
Before their nations, their lands, their bodies.
Before their tattooed heads, their skins
their vaginas, penises and wombs,
were smashed into millions of fragmented pieces
Before they were disembowelled
Disembodied
Reduced to collectable artefacts,
Exotic furnishings for the salons and siting rooms
Of the wealthy
The process of dehumanising,
Of not recognising the human
Of rendering others as beasts of burden
As less than human
As partial humans
As not quite humans
As soul less beings
As savage creatures
The process of conquering the Other
Of wielding them to the will of empires
Is deeply written in the history of Europe
Of Rome and Greece
Of Great Britain
Of Versailles
Of little fiefdoms and all conquering heroes
We read in Europe's history of itself
The separation of flora and fauna,
Of humans from others beings
Of humans from nature
Of mind and body
Of white and black
Of civilised and savage
The positing of a soul, heaven and hell,
Of human will, intelligence, morality
Of emotions
Of race
Of gender

Of the being of a human
Of the rights of a human
Of the natural order of things
These were the technologies that
Were present and were honed
in the colonies
In the Concentration Camps
In the prisons
On the reserves
In the laboratories
In the institutions of knowledge
These are the tools we teach\and promote
That will inform
And discipline
That will help
And save
That will develop
And advance
The humans that these tools have dehumanised
The stories that these tools have silenced
The relationships that these tools have subverted
The environment that these tools have contaminated
It began in the foment of language and ideas
Incited by power and opportunity
Emboldened by a sense of Godliness
Institutionalised in Church and State
Practised on women
On children
On the poor
On other human beings
It was taken with the WORD
And the SWORD
Across oceans.
And continents,
Across mountains
And deserts and rivers
It was present in their gaze as they surveyed
The land of others
It was present in their bodies as they
Infected villages, cities and civilisations
It was present in their minds
As they built their governments, missions and schools
As they made laws and regulations

As they built prisons and slums
Laboratories and roads.
Their values
Their beliefs
Their norms
Their words
Their feelings
Their touch
Their thoughts
Their fears
Their dreams
Their fantasies
It began there
In the essence of their humanity.

## Renewing

Selma Sevenhuijsen (2003) pointed the way to using the ethics of care not only to critique but also to renew policy with care. In this book we have tried to do something similar in relation to research. One thing that is needed as we research together is a care-full tact that enables people to work together in a way that values the contribution that different people make to the research. Haraway (2016) refers to rendering the other as capable to enable practices with companions – including the pigeons we named in Chapter 4. The tact that this requires involves the ability to create interstices, spaces, time for catching up and getting to know each other. Knowing the conditions of each other's lives can influence how people are able to be with each other and to relate to each other with care. This may include identifying difference, or disagreements, which are further chances to engage to understand differently. Caring for each other through this process is paramount in our approach as it is keenly felt when care is not present. This is our interdependence. Recognising our own emotional reactions to experiences of care or lack of care can also raise the need for us to look after ourselves, and this raises the possibility that others may also be struggling with the experience. Locating emotional responses in the self and discussing them opens a discussion about the need for care when it may not be present. Our hope is that the stories people have told to us will help others see how this can be possible in the work they do together.

People tell stories in many ways. From an ethics of care perspective, creating the space and allowing people the time to tell the story is attentiveness in action. In research with people with dementia, for example, telling the story may be a collective effort over multiple visits, with prompts like photographs or other memorabilia. The point from A to B is not always straightforward and increasingly innovative and creative approaches are used to enable people to share, including, for example, the use of diaries, photographs, poetry or theatre. Bourgault (2016) warns us against non-listening in busy lives. Here, Hughes-Warrington, a historian interested in ethical histories, reflects on listening to Aunty Anne Martin, an Aboriginal rights activist and educator, in conversation:

> Aunty Anne talks in circles. Big and little ones, beautiful and incomplete. They intersect and encircle past, present, herself and the world and me. They also leap, weave and ripple, sometimes plunging with the force of a muttonfish (Abalone) diver and sometimes dancing like fingers tracing the surface of tidal sands. The first time I heard her speak, I struggled to make sense. I searched for a linear order, a spatio-temporal scale to slide up and down, a before and an after, a cause, and its ethical effects. The shortest point between two lines. All the while, her laughing eyes and enfolding stories looped history around me, and she reeled me in. (Hughes-Warrington and Martin, 2022, p 187)

In many contexts researchers have needed to learn patient listening when 'respondents' veer off the point, recount anecdotes that we can't immediately understand as connected with the question we have posed. In our conversation with her, Bunty talked about one of the members of the older people's research team who would often do this and the different responses this generated among team members. The frustration that this can engender among some suggests a need for a much better focus on attentiveness as a research skill. In Pacific research, in this case Tongan, *talanoa* is an acceptable way of getting together to explore and talk through an issue of importance to the community. It is expected to take some time because it is important to ensure that people are able to contribute in the way that they want to and that some themes are agreed within the group before it ends (Vaka et al, 2016).

One of the themes that came through in the conversations we had with the people who contributed to the book, is the attention needed about the process of doing research together, the creation of space for people to share and the creativity this engenders. Rather than frustration at irrelevance, we need to listen and open ourselves to the possibility of new understanding. Others have written about this in different ways. Anna Tsing (2015) has written about this as the *contaminations* that occur as different perspectives mingle. Donna Haraway (2016) discussed collaborations that generate *composts* through learning together. We might suggest that what we and others experience are the sometimes unexpected consequences of the threads of different lives being woven together, not following a predetermined pattern, but mixing to produce textures and patterns that would not have been possible had all the threads been of the same colour and ply. Sometimes this can involve provocations. Nerves may be touched, some may feel discomfort at the lack of an established plan or be unsettled by the adjustments that are necessary. Some are energised by their own assumptions being challenged, confronted or refuted, while others are reassured by validations of what they can contribute and their capacity to name what was unnamed. Kearney (in O'Rourke, 2018) writes of a hospitality of narratives where contributions are viewed as a gift from one to another to create an openness to receiving stories, for example from conflict or war. Kearney notes that Jacques Derrida coined the term *hostipitality*, because such gifts can be experienced as either care or hostility. So we need to be careful about this. Taking care of the people and making space for exchange is at the heart of ethics of care research. We can learn a lot from indigenous processes of setting and nurturing new relationships. The care that we extend through research partnerships needs to be politically aware and sensitive to the experiences of all, bearing in mind that the process of participation can generate unexpected responses. The purpose of these entanglements is to be together, to learn together and to transform ourselves and each other. This is an exposure of selves, of experiences, of positions, of ontologies, and provides the richness we seek in the doing of research. Transformations occur in small and simple steps that eventually lead to revolutions (Robinson, 2015).

## Reflections on doing research with ethics of care

*Marian*

> Once you have become a feminist, it can feel that you were
> always a feminist.
>
> Ahmed, 2017, p 6

To me, it also feels like that in terms of care ethics. Having 'discovered' this work, having recognised the way in which thinking with care spoke to discomforts; revealed things that were suppressed; offered a language; an intellectual and political respectability for saying things that felt hard to say, it feels like this way of thinking about the world and my place in it, was always there. This is why Gilligan's analysis of the silencing that girls and women experience is so powerful. Part of who I am is to try to think the world, my relationships with other people, with the environment and non-human animals, with the relational insights of care ethics. I try to act with care, and I feel uncomfortable when I acknowledge how hard this is and how I get it wrong. But thinking with care enables me to be more attentive, to myself and others, and not to resist what my emotional responses tell me about what matters. I recognise that, both personally and politically, neither I nor others can do justice without care. I have revisited some of my earlier work to reflect on it from a care ethics perspective, both in the obvious context of reflecting on the experiences of family carers (Barnes, 2006) and the perhaps less obvious context of analyses of deliberative democracy (Barnes, 2008, 2019b). And I have recognised the necessity of connecting the personal and the professional.

One thing that struck me during work researching with old people is the force of the dynamic intersections in our lives. The intersectional self is a self that is always becoming. When I write about the project on old people and wellbeing now, when I am older than some of those who took part both as interviewees and as those we called 'older co-researchers', I live the reality that older people are our future selves and I question the way that I name those others. As we grow older material shifts – bodily changes and loss of physical capacities; status changes – from senior professional to retired person; as well as the loss of people close to us – intersect with the way we are viewed by and the responses we evoke from others. The social, cultural and political changes taking place around us can leave us unsettled and feeling out of place and time. If we are to thrive throughout change we need a sense of being a part of something beyond ourselves, a movement or movements, a set of values or commitments that hold us together with others (Barnes, 2018). It can feel even more important to feel solidarity with others who are different from ourselves: who are younger; from different cultural backgrounds; differently positioned in relation to care; living in conditions of greater poverty, environmental or violent threats, with experiences of racism or other oppressions. Feminist care ethics offers a way of making sense of how we can live well together that invites solidarities across these differences and that invites us to explore what connections can be like when we reach out beyond the usual and familiar.

Among the specific contexts in which I have been rethinking my life post-retirement, what it means to live well in the world and to seek to repair harms, has been encounters with a Christian residential community. I am not a Christian and for most of my life religion has not been a relevant consideration. I simply had no contact with it, it did not enter my sphere of attention. If I did think about it, it was to reinforce my puzzlement as to how people could believe in a god or in life after death. My disbelief was not helped by evidence of abuses within parts of the Christian church. I still do not share the faith, I still despair of how some manage to reconcile a god of love with violence and abuse. But having now spent extended periods of time living with others in a community founded and sustained by members who profess a Christian faith, I have developed respect for and experienced solidarity with those for whom faith is the basis on which they care for others who live with pain and brokenness in their lives, and who live in a sustainable way with the animals and land that nurtures their lives together (Barnes et al, 2022). It has been an example of an unexpected boundary to reach across in order to live care in a different way. And I was glad to have the opportunity to deepen my understanding through researching the community with others involved in it.

For me, encountering this community intersected with increasing awareness of the damage inflicted on the world by ways of life that regard the other-than-human world as a resource to be exploited. As well as injustices based in age, disability or mental illness that had been the focus of much of my research, I have become more attentive to the unjust consequences of changes to the climate and to indigenous ways of life consequent on the imperialism of western capitalism. In the face of existential crises of climate change and pandemic, evidence of small ways in which living life with care can achieve small, but significant, transformations feel vital to sustaining hope. When I see evidence of the enduring distrust consequent on unethical research such as the Tuskegee studies we cited in Chapter 3, impacting the willingness of Black Americans to receive COVID-19 vaccinations (This Body/Black America, hope, trust and COVID-19 vaccination trials[1]), I know the importance of researching with care. How we research leaves a legacy that extends beyond that of which we are aware. So we do what we can in those spaces we have access to. Recognising research as one of the things we do that has an impact on the way in which we can live together in the world as well as possible is necessary for all of us who care about and accept responsibility for the way in which our approach to knowledge generation can contribute to social justice. Once you have embraced feminist care ethics it feels like you have tried to live it throughout your life.

## Tula

Care ethics and research coincided during my PhD study, and it was Marian that introduced Selma Sevenhuijsen's (1998) book to me. At that point, I had been a mental health nurse for 13 years, having trained at an old asylum hospital. My colleagues and I witnessed a catalogue of human rights abuses during our training, and throughout practice I was constantly questioning, challenging and occasionally whistleblowing the standards of care I thought were poor. I found my niche working with older people with mental health challenges and dementia as it gave me autonomy to care well, and I moved away from the practices that I found particularly troubling. Studying research methods at university was a lightbulb moment about the possibilities of being able to design and carry out research to improve practice. My first undergraduate study looked at the adoption of cultures of care in nursing homes for people with dementia, which means that I examined whether people were treated as people or as objects. When I read Sevenhuijsen and Tronto my immediate reaction was to question why I did not know this as a practitioner. It provides a different way of understanding the aims of care, a language to explain the shortfalls of what was achieved in practice, a guide or a review of decision making in situations where there is conflict between families and the treating team, and in practice, there were a fair few of these that felt fundamentally problematic. These included families wanting medical interventions such as tube feeding for people no longer able to swallow and at the very last stages of dementia, or stopping active treatment for a woman so distressed she cried and screamed all day. I teach ethics of care to undergraduate students and postgraduate practitioners to provide helpful ways of thinking and talking about ethics and care.

In research, my first use of the ethics of care was as an analytical technique to examine the decisions of practitioners when considering participation in decision making about residential placement for people with dementia. Care ethics has permeated my thinking. Every dilemma or problem that I encounter is thought through with an ethics of care. I can't see the world without thinking about care. Two aspects of care ethics particularly speak to this and unsurprisingly they are care deficit and recognising that care is sometimes not care (Tronto 1993, 2013). The care deficit acknowledges that the people in the most need of care, receive the least care. Think of a disabled person living alone who gets two calls for 30 minutes per day and contrast that to the person who has a personal assistant to help arrange their schedule, a nanny for the children, a cleaner for the house and carers for any other dependents. It is wrong that the world is arranged in such a way that this is normed in some societies. Joan Tronto (1993) also called for care that is not care to be recognised as such. Colonisation was not care, institutionalisation was not care. In research, there is the opportunity to work alongside people to make reparations about what has happened in their world, and I would argue that some of the best recovery work I have done with people who have used mental health services is not located in practice, but in research partnerships where people can use their knowledge for a different purpose, one that is infused with ideas of social justice and change.

In research, the ethics of care is a constant guide to analysis of care and the analysis of practices, including my own. I am now settled back in Aotearoa New Zealand, my adopted home where I am very grateful to the *manu whenua* (people of the land) for their hospitality to host me here. I expected an engagement in indigenous–settler relations but have been enlivened by adopting an ally position to support decolonisation, albeit from my clumsy *tauiwi* (foreigner) position. I have written elsewhere about the potential of the ethics of care to support research practices that are acceptable and sensitive to Māori in order to work together to make changes that create a different future for the next generation. I hope this book makes a contribution for new researchers to strengthen their commitment to working well in their research.

I would like to thank the people who we spoke to for this book for their contributions and here reflect on what was informative about those conversations. Bea enlightened me about the ongoing relational care with Marian and Bunty, but also about how ethics of care influenced her personally in her roles outside of that partnership. Everything was better when done in partnership, and the sum of two parts made more than the whole in terms of the effects on many more people than the research touched. Bea's reaction to knowing the ethics of care inside and out resonated deeply with me. Bea also talked of the huge joy of the work and how to communicate that joy to others not connected to the research. The conversation with Ceri resonated for our shared experiences working with indigenous people, and the efforts not to offend. In the conversation with Ceri there was a sense of circling to get somewhere, a gradual building towards something, and this resonated too, by which we develop and transform ourselves. Ceri and I talked of a 'baptism of Whiteness', a need to understand how Whiteness operates to provides privilege, as a signal to others and how to counter that or dispel assumptions that others hold. It all means something, it may be that hindsight helps us understand it. Ceri and Ruth brought to our attention the importance of care for all in the team and how to formalise this in funding bids, processes and protocols and making sure it is very much on the radar of the research project. Umut's work is unequivocally concerned with some of the most marginalised people in the UK and unapologetically reframes and deliberates the conditions of life for these groups with an intention of changing the conversation. Umut shows a level of attention to detail that constantly refines definitions and pulls the focus back to the ethical place it should be and this is a dedicated and committed position of constant reinforcement. And Viv reminded me about the challenge that can be laid in the everyday work we do as academics in terms of creating a different conversation and opening spaces for new voices in the academy. Lastly, I would like to reflect on Joan Tronto's contribution to this book as Joan prompted the thinking for this book at a conference in Prague in November 2017, where in a discussion after Joan's presentation on caring democracies, she suggested that while ethics of care was burgeoning in novel disciplines, not much attention had been given to the application of ethics of care thinking to research. I took this as a call to action that built on the thinking I had done in applying the feminist ethics of care to research partnerships with Māori.

## Horizon scanning

Horizon scanning using the ethics of care enables us to consider what supports research with care, for us to identify what we see as facilitative or contentious to doing research with care. Donna Haraway (2016) describes the period we are currently in as the Chthulucene, in which post-disciplinarity and interspecies research approaches that are cognisant of environmental impacts are valued. Robin Wall Kimmerer (2020) similarly calls for research that acknowledges the gifts the earth offers and aims to reciprocate in kind, showing love to the earth and its people. The work that we do happens in place and has an impact on that place, on the current and future people of that place, and, to use Haraway's term, the critters there. Research needs to acknowledge the resources used in its process and to contribute to rather than deplete those resources. Deb McGregor calls for research that shows love for future generations, and we would call for this to be integrated as a key question for research – how it contributes to make a better future. These approaches are consistent with Tronto's (2013) definition of care that seeks care and repair for the world as we exist in it. Iris Marion Young's (2011) connection of the ethic of responsibility with the ethics of research speaks about the way in which we are implicated for injustices even if we have not directly acted in an unjust way. This is very relevant when working in contexts of racism, colonisation and other oppressions.

It is to be expected that research attracts people who have a healthy distrust of institutions or governmental departments, who want to ask critical questions, are keen to change and repair the world. In spite of the promise of participatory research, researchers question the extent of transformation that this has achieved (Mocarski et al, 2020). Wykes (2014) and Mocarski et al (2020) identified that methodologies that were inclusive of people with experience have not achieved a paradigm shift and not much has changed in the material conditions of life for marginalised communities. There is potential for paradigm shift to come from researching with care if this encompasses not only the process of research, but also the ways in which research is funded and reviewed, and the priorities that are implemented with regard to legacies that support responsibility for action. The particular moment in which we have been writing much of this book has necessitated reflection on other fundamental questions. Not only have we, the book's authors, been unable to meet face to face to discuss it, neither have researchers been able to conduct face to face work for much of this time. While online research is convenient and here to stay, it is not adequate to accommodate initial stages of relational care so that people may participate as well as possible.

As well as impacting how we research, care ethicists, along with many others, have highlighted how social and political inequalities have played out through the health inequities of the COVID-19 pandemic, both within nations and internationally (Gary and Berlinger, 2020), which deserves a critical and intersectional analysis (Williams, 2021). How we seek to influence future practices to prevent both the occurrence and unequal impact of future pandemics will depend, in part, on how we go about researching what happened and why in relation to COVID-19. Our entanglements and interdependencies with the more-than-human world cannot be ignored.

The necessity for collaborations across disciplines and between those who identify as researchers and those who see themselves as practitioners in other fields is ever more visible. Having an open and inquisitive approach helps draw out the knowledge that can inform us, to ask the difficult and challenging questions that can bring about meaningful change. Only through good relational care and creative spaces can these challenges be explored.

On a final note, we would like to extend our encouragement to people using ethics of care to guide and review research practices. The feminist origins and intentions of the ethics of care are well explicated in Gilligan and Tronto's work and it is this work we have intentionally used to develop ethics of care research to preserve this feminist commitment. The feminist commitment is to recognition, responsibility and solidarity, and we have argued that these elements are necessary for care ethics to have its transformational potential. Researching with care is intended to inform the radical potential of a different politics.

# Notes

## Chapter 3

[1] Examples include accounts recorded by the Shaping Our Lives project, and by the Survivors History Group: www.shapingourlives.org.uk and www.studymore.org.uk.

## Chapter 4

[1] https://multispeciesdementia.org/.

[2] Ceri Davies was one of the researchers we spoke with for this book and more insights from her work are included in Part II.

[3] Details of this project and the art generated from it can be found at www.olderpeople selffundingcare.com.

## Chapter 8

[1] This Body/Black America, hope, trust and COVID-19 vaccination trials, Guardian video at www.theguardian.com/global/video/2021/jul/29/this-body-black-america-hope-trust-and-covid-vaccine-trials-video.

# References

Abah, O.S. and Okwori, J.Z. (2005) 'A nation in search of citizens: Problems of citizenship in the Nigerian context' in N. Kabeer (ed) *Inclusive Citizenship: Meanings and Expressions*, London: Zed Books, pp 71–84.

Ahmed, S. (2017) *Living a Feminist Life*, Durham, NC: Duke University Press.

Alzheimer Europe Report (2015) *Ethical Dilemmas Faced by Health and Social Care Professionals Providing Dementia Care in Care Homes and Hospital Settings: A Guide for Use in the Context of Ongoing Professional Care Training*, Luxembourg: Alzheimer Europe, www.alzheimer-europe.org/Publications/Alzheimer-Europe-Reports

Banks, S., Hart, A., Pahl, K. and Ward, P. (eds) (2018) *Co-Producing Research: A Community Development Approach*, Bristol: Policy Press.

Banks, S., Cook, T., Kong, S.T. and Stavropolou, N. (2019) 'Brushed under the carpet: Examining the complexities of participatory research', *Research for All*, 3(2), 161–79.

Barber, R., Boote, J., Parry, G., Cooper, C. and Yeeles, P. (2012) 'Evaluating the impact of public involvement in research' in M. Barnes and P. Cotterell (eds) *Critical Perspectives on User Involvement*, Bristol: Policy Press, pp 217–23.

Barker, P., Campbell, P. and Davidson, B. (eds) (1999) *From the Ashes of Experience: Reflections on Madness, Survival and Growth*, London: Whurr Publishers.

Barnes, C. and Mercer, G. (eds) (1997) *Doing Disability Research*, Leeds: Leeds Disability Press, University of Leeds.

Barnes, M. (2002) 'Bringing difference into deliberation: Disabled people, survivors and local governance', *Policy and Politics*, 30(3), 355–368.

Barnes, M. (2006) *Caring and Social Justice*, Basingstoke: Palgrave.

Barnes, M. (2008) 'Passionate participation: Emotional experiences and expressions in deliberative forums', *Critical Social Policy*, 28(4), 461–481.

Barnes, M. (2011) 'Abandoning care? A critical perspective on personalisation from an ethic of care', *Ethics and Social Welfare*, 5(2), 153–167.

Barnes, M. (2015) 'Survivors, consumers or experts by experience? Assigned, chosen and contested identities in the mental health service user movement' in A. McGarry and J.M. Jasper (eds) *The Identity Dilemma: Social Movements and Collective Identity*, Philadelphia: Temple University Press, pp 131–49.

Barnes, M. (2018) 'Getting out of line: Reflections on ageing activism and moral agency', *Ethics and Social Welfare*, 12(3), 204–215.

Barnes, M. (2019a) 'Community care: The ethics of care in a residential community', *Ethics and Social Welfare*, 14(2), 140–155.

Barnes, M. (2019b) 'Old age and caring democracy' in H. Tam (ed) *Whose Government Is It? The Renewal of State-Citizen Cooperation*, Bristol: Policy Press, pp 143–58.

Barnes, M. and Cotterell, P. (eds) (2012) *Critical Perspectives on User Involvement*, Bristol: Policy Press.

Barnes, M. and Henwood, F. (2015) 'Inform with care: Ethics and information in care for people with dementia', *Ethics and Social Welfare*, 9(2), 147–163.

Barnes, M. and Prior, D. (eds) (2009) *Subversive Citizens: Power, Agency and Resistance in Public Services*, Bristol: Policy Press.

Barnes, M., Harrison, S., Mort, M. and Shardlow, P. (1999) *Unequal Partners: User Groups and Community Care*, Bristol: Policy Press.

Barnes, M., Davis, A. and Tew, J. (2000) 'Valuing experience: Users' experiences of compulsion under the Mental Health Act 1983', *The Mental Health Review*, 5(3), 11–14.

Barnes, M., Bauld, L., Benzeval, M., Judge, K., Mackenzie, M. and Sullivan, H. (2005) *Health Action Zones: Partnerships for Health Equity*, London: Routledge.

Barnes, M., Brannelly, T., Ward, L. and Ward, N. (2015) *Ethics of Care: Critical Advances in International Perspectives*, Bristol: Policy Press.

Barnes, M., Gahagan, B. and Ward, L. (2018) *Re-imagining Old Age: Wellbeing, Care and Participation*, Wilmington, DE: Vernon Press.

Barnes, M., Davies, M. and Prior, D. (2022) *Living Life in Common: Stories from the Pilsdon Community*, Leicester: Matador.

Bartlett, R. (2014) 'Citizenship in action: The lived experiences of citizens with dementia who campaign for social change', *Disability & Society*, 29(8), 1291–304.

Bartlett, R. and Brannelly, T. (2018) *Life at Home for People with a Dementia*, London: Routledge.

Bartlett, R. and Brannelly, T. (2020) 'On being outdoors: How people with dementia experience and deal with vulnerabilities', *Social Science and Medicine*, 235.

Beresford, P. (2002) 'User involvement in research and evaluation: Liberation or regulation?', *Social Policy and Society*, 1(2), 95–105.

Beresford, P. and Branfield, F. (2012) 'Building solidarity, ensuring diversity: Lessons from service users' and disabled people's movements' in M. Barnes and P. Cotterell (eds) *Critical Perspectives on User Involvement*, Bristol: Policy Press, pp 217–233.

Boulton, A. and Brannelly, T. (2015) 'Care ethics and indigenous values: Political, tribal and personal', in M. Barnes, T. Brannelly, L. Ward and L. Ward (eds) *Ethics of Care: Critical Advances in International Perspective*, Bristol: Policy Press, pp 69–82.

Bourgault, S. (2016) 'Attentive listening and care in a neoliberal era: Weilian insights for hurried times', *Etica & Politica / Ethics & Politics*, 18(3), 311–337.

Bozalek, V. (2015) 'Privilege and responsibility in the South African context', in M. Barnes, T. Brannelly, L. Ward and N. Ward (eds) *Ethics of Care: Critical Advances in International Perspectives*, Bristol: Policy Press.

Bozalek, V. and Zembylas, M. (2017) 'Diffraction or reflection? Sketching the contours of two methodologies in educational research', *International Journal of Qualitative Studies in Education*, 30(2), 111–127.

Bozalek, V., Bayat, A., Motala, S., Mitchell, V. and Gachago, D. (2016) 'Diffracting socially just pedagogies through stained glass', *South African Journal of Higher Education*, 30(3), 201–218.

Bozalek, V., Zembylas, M., Motala, S. and Holscher, D. (eds) (2021) *Higher Education Hauntologies: Living with Ghosts for a Justice-to-Come*, London: Routledge.

Brady, L.-M., Davis, E., Ghosh, A., Surti, B. and Wilson, L. (2012) 'Involving young people in research: Making an impact in public health' in M. Barnes and P. Cotterell (eds) *Critical Perspectives on User Involvement*, Bristol: Policy Press, pp 159–168.

Brannelly, P. (2006) 'Negotiating ethics in dementia care', *Dementia*, 5(2), 197–212.

Brannelly, T. (2011) 'That others matter: The moral achievement – care ethics and citizenship in practice with people with dementia', *Ethics and Social Welfare*, 5(2), 210–216.

Brannelly, T. (2016) 'Citizenship and people living with dementia: A case for the ethics of care', *Dementia*, 15(3), 304–314.

Brannelly, T. (2018) 'An ethics of care research manifesto', *International Journal of Care and Caring*, 2(3), 367–378.

Brannelly, T. and Bartlett, R. (2021) 'Using walking interviews to enhance research relations with people with dementia: Methodological insights from an empirical study conducted in England', *Ethics and Social Welfare*, 14(4), 432–442.

Brannelly, T. and Boulton, A. (2017) 'The ethics of care and transformational research practices in Aotearoa New Zealand', *Qualitative Research*, 17(3), 340–350.

Brannelly, T., Boulton, A. and Te Hiini, A. (2013a) 'A relationship between the ethics of care and Māori worldview: The place of relationality and care in Maori mental health service provision', *Ethics and Social Welfare*, 7(4), 410–422.

Brannelly, T., Boulton, A. and Wilson, S. (2013b) 'Developing citizens: Missed opportunities in health and social care provision? A view from Aotearoa New Zealand', *Child & Youth Services*, 34(3), 218–235.

Brett, J., Staniszewska, S., Mockford, C., Herron-Marx, S., Hughes, J., Tysall, C. and Suleman, R. (2014) 'Mapping the impact of patient and public involvement on health and social care research: A systematic review', *Health Expectations*, 17(5), 637–50.

Brown, J. (2018) 'Dilemmas of disclosure in mental health therapeutic education' in J. Wintrup, H. Biggs, T. Brannelly, A. Fenwick, A. Ingham and D. Woods (eds) *Ethics from the Ground Up: Emerging Debates, Changing Practices and New Voices in Healthcare*, Basingstoke: Palgrave Macmillan, pp 32–44.

Brown, P. (1998) 'Shaping the evaluator's role in a theory of change evaluation' in K. Fulbright-Anderson, A.C. Kubisch and J.P. Connell (eds) *New Approaches to Evaluating Community Initiatives, Vol. 2: Theory, Measurement and Analysis*, Washington, DC: The Aspen Institute.

Campbell, J. and Oliver, M. (1996) *Disability Politics: Understanding Our Past, Changing Our Future*, London: Routledge.

Church, K. (2004) *Forbidden Narratives: Critical Autobiography as Social Science*, London: Routledge.

Clarke, C., Wilkinson, H., Watson, J., Wilcockson, J., Kinnaird, L. and Williamson, T. (2018a) 'A seat around the table: Participatory data analysis with people living with dementia', *Qualitative Health Research*, 28(9), 1421–1433.

Clarke, C., Wilcockson, J., Watson, J., Wilkinson, H., Keyes, S., Kinnaird, L. and Williamson, T. (2018b) 'Relational care and co-operative endeavour: Reshaping dementia care through participatory secondary data analysis', *Dementia*, 19(4), 1151–1172.

Clarke, S., Hoggett, P. and Thompson, S. (eds) (2006) *Emotion, Politics and Society*, Basingstoke: Palgrave.

Clifford, D. (2019) 'Deficits in health and social care research ethics: A personal perspective', *Ethics and Social Welfare*, 13(4), 434–437.

Collins, S. (2015) *The Core of Care Ethics*, Basingstoke: Palgrave Macmillan.

Connell, J.P., Kubisch, A., Schorr, C., Lisbeth, B. and Weiss, C.H. (eds) (1995) *New Approaches to Evaluating Community Initiatives: Concepts, Methods and Contexts*, Washington, DC: The Aspen Institute.

Connelly, S., Vanderhoven, D., Durose, C., Matthews, P., Richardson, L. and Rutherford, R. (2017) 'Translation across borders: Connecting the academic and policy communities' in K. Facer and K. Pahl (eds) *Valuing Interdisciplinary Collaborative Research: Beyond Impact*, Bristol: Policy Press, pp 173–189.

Criado Perez, C. (2018) *Invisible Women: Exposing Data Bias in a World Designed for Men*, London: Vintage.

Cunningham, M. (2012) 'The apology in politics' in S. Thompson and P. Hoggett (eds) *Politics and the Emotions: The Affective Turn in Contemporary Political Studies*, London: Continuum, pp 139–156.

Dalmiya, V. (2016) *Caring to Know: Comparative Care Ethics, Feminist Epistemology, and the Mahābhārata*, Oxford Scholarship Online, doi:10.1093/acprof:oso/9780199464760.001.0001.

Davey, B. (1994) 'Madness and its causative contexts', *Changes, International Journal of Psychology and Psychotherapy*, 12(2), pp 113–131.

Davies, C.J. (2016) *Whose Knowledge Counts? Exploring Cognitive Justice in Community-University Collaborations*, thesis, University of Brighton.

Desai, K. and Sanya, B.N. (2016) 'Towards decolonial praxis: Reconfiguring the human and curriculum', *Gender and Education*, 28(6), 710–724.

Edwards, R. and Brannelly, T. (2017) 'Approaches to democratising qualitative research methods', *Qualitative Research*, 17(3), 271–277.

Edwards, R., Barnes, H., McGregor, D. and Brannelly, T. (2020) 'Supporting Indigenous and non-Indigenous research partnerships', *The Qualitative Report*, 25(13), 6–15.

Erel, U. (2018) 'Saving and reproducing the nation: Struggles around right-wing politics of social reproduction, gender and race in austerity Europe', *Women's Studies International Forum*, 68, 173–182.

Erel, U., Reynolds, T. and Kaptani, E. (2017) 'Participatory theatre for transformative social research', *Qualitative Research*, 17(3), 302–312.

Erel, U., Reynolds, T. and Kaptani, E. (2018) 'Migrant mothers creative interventions into racialised citizenships', *Ethnic and Racial Studies*, 41(1), 55–72.

Evans, R. (2014) 'Parental death as a vital conjuncture? Intergenerational care and responsibility following bereavement in Senegal', *Social & Cultural Geography*, 15(5), 547–570.

Evans, R. (2015) 'Negotiating intergenerational relations and care in diverse African contexts' in R. Vanderbeck and N. Worth (eds) *Intergenerational Space*, London: Routledge, pp 199–213.

Evans, R. (2019) 'Interpreting family struggles in West Africa across majority-minority world boundaries: Tensions and possibilities', *Gender, Place & Culture*. doi:10.1080/0966369X.2018.1553861.

Evans, R. and Becker, S. (2009) *Children Caring for Parents with HIV and AIDS: Global Issues and Policy Responses*, Bristol: Policy Press.

Evans, R., Ribbens McCarthy, J., Kébé, F., Bowlby, S. and Wouango, J. (2017) 'Interpreting "grief" in Senegal: Language, emotions and cross-cultural translation in a Francophone African context', *Mortality*, 22(2), 118–135.

Facer, K. and Pahl, K. (eds) (2017) *Valuing Interdisciplinary Collaborative Research: Beyond Impact*, Bristol: Policy Press.

Faulkner, A. and Tallis, D. (2009) 'Survivor research: Ethics approval and ethical practice' in A. Sweeney, P. Beresford, A. Faulkner, M. Nettle and D. Rose (eds) *This is Survivor Research*, Ross on Wye: PCCS Books, pp 53–62.

Figert, A.E. (1996) *Women and the Ownership of PMS: The Structuring of a Psychiatric Disorder*, New York: Aldine de Gruyter.

Fricker, M. (2007) *Epistemic Injustice: Power and the Ethics of Knowing*, Oxford: Oxford University Press.

Gary, M. and Berlinger, N. (2020) Interdependent citizens: The ethics of care in pandemic recovery, *Hastings Centre Report*, May–June, 50(3), 56–58.

Gilligan, C. (1982) *In a Different Voice*, Cambridge, MA: Harvard University Press.

Gilligan, C. (1993) *In a Different Voice*, 2nd edn, Cambridge, MA: Harvard University Press.

Gilligan, C. (2011) *Joining the Resistance*, Cambridge: Polity Press.

Gilroy, P., Sandset, T., Bangstad, S. and Ringen Høibjerg, G. (2019) 'A diagnosis of contemporary forms of racism, race and nationalism: A conversation with Professor Paul Gilroy', *Cultural Studies*, 33(2), 173–197.

Godfrey, M. (ed) (2019) *Olafur Eliasson in Real Life*, London: Tate.

Goodwin, J., Jasper, J.M. and Polletta, F. (eds) (2001) *Passionate Politics: Emotions and Social Movements*, Chicago: University of Chicago Press.

Gould, D.B. (2012) 'Political despair' in S. Thompson and P. Hoggett (eds) *Politics and the Emotions: The Affective Turn in Contemporary Political Studies*, London: Continuum, pp 95–114.

Hajer, M.A. and Wagenaar, H. (eds) (2003) *Deliberative Policy Analysis*, Cambridge: Cambridge University Press.

Hamington, M. (2018) 'Care, competency and knowledge' in M. Visse and T. Abma (eds) *Evaluation for a Caring Society*, Charlotte, NC: Information Age Publishing.

Hamington, M. and Rosenow, C. (2019) *Care Ethics and Poetry*, Cham: Palgrave/Springer.

Haraway, D. (2016) *Staying with the Trouble: Making Kin in the Chthulucene*, Durham, NC: Duke University Press.

Held, V. (2006) *The Ethics of Care: Personal, Political and Global*, Oxford: Oxford University Press.

Hoggett, P. (2006) 'Pity, compassion, solidarity' in S. Clarke, P. Hoggett and S. Thompson (eds) *Emotion, Politics and Society*, Basingstoke: Palgrave, pp 145–61.

Honneth, A. (1996) *The Struggle for Recognition: The Moral Grammar of Social Conflicts*, Cambridge: Polity Press.

Hudson, M., Milne, M., Reynolds, P., Russell, K. and Smith, B. (2010) *Te Ara Tika, Guidelines for Māori Research Ethics: A Framework for Researchers and Ethics Committee Members*, Wellington: Health Research Council.

Hughes-Warrington, M. and Martin, A. (2022) *Big and Little Histories: Sizing Up Ethics in Historiography*, London: Routledge.

Hunter, S. (2015) *Power, Politics and the Emotions: Impossible Governance?*, Abingdon: Routledge.

Kara, H. and Khoo, S.M. (2020a) *Researching in the Age of COVID-19 Volume I: Response and Reassessment*, Bristol: Policy Press.

Kara, H. and Khoo, S.M. (2020b) *Researching in the Age of COVID-19 Volume II: Care and Resilience*, Bristol: Policy Press.

Kara, H. and Khoo, S.M. (2020c) *Researching in the Age of COVID-19 Volume III: Creativity and Ethics*, Bristol: Policy Press.

Kidd, J., Came, J.H., Herbert, S. and McCreanor, T. (2020) 'Māori and tauiwi nurses' perspectives of anti-racist praxis: Findings from a qualitative pilot study', *AlterNative*, 16(4), 387–394.

Kimmerer, R.W. (2020) *Braiding Sweetgrass: Indigenous Wisdom, Scientific Knowledge and the Teachings of Plants*, New York: Penguin Random House.

Kittay, E.F. (2010) 'The personal is philosophical is political: A philosopher and mother of a cognitively disabled person sends notes from the battlefield' in E.F. Kittay and L. Carlson (eds) *Cognitive Disability and its Challenge to Moral Philosophy*, Chichester: Wiley-Blackwell, pp 393–413.

Kittay, E.F. (2015) 'A theory of justice as fair terms of social life given our inevitable dependency and our inextricable interdependency' in D. Engster and M. Hamington (eds) *Care Ethics and Political Theory*, Oxford Scholarship Online, doi: 10.1093/acp rof:oso/9780198716341.001.0001.

Kuhn, T.S. (1970) *The Structure of Scientific Revolutions*, 2nd edn, Chicago: University of Chicago Press.

Kutchins, H. and Kirk, S.A. (1997) *Making Us Crazy: DSM – the Psychiatric Bible and the Creation of Mental Disorders*, London: Constable.

Langford, R. (ed) (2019) *Theorizing Feminist Ethics of Care in Early Childhood Practice*, London: Bloomsbury Academic.

Leibowitz, B. and Bozalek, V. (2016) 'The scholarship of teaching and learning from a social justice perspective', *Teaching in Higher Education*, 21(2), 109–122.

Letherby, G. (2003) *Feminist Research in Theory and Practice*, Buckingham: Open University Press.

Levac, L., Ronis, S., Cowper-Smith, Y. and Vaccarino, O. (2019) 'A scoping review: The utility of participatory research approaches in psychology', *Journal of Community Psychology*, 47(8), 1865–1892.

Lewis-Stempel, J. (2016) *The Running Hare: The Secret Life of Farmland*, London: Penguin Random House.

Lloyd, L. (2010) 'The individual in social care: The ethics of care and the "personalisation" agenda in services for older people in England', *Ethics and Social Welfare*, 4(2), 188–200.

Mackay, F. (2001) *Love and Politics: Women Politicians and the Ethics of Care*, London: Continuum.

Mason, P. and Barnes, M. (2007) 'Constructing theories of change: Methods and sources', *Evaluation*, 13(2), 151–170.

McGarry, A. and Jasper, J.M. (eds) (2015) *The Identity Dilemma: Social Movements and Collective Identity*, Philadelphia: Temple University Press.

McGregor, D., Restoule, J.P. and Johnson, R. (eds) (2018) *Indigenous Research: Theories, Practices, and Relationships*, Toronto: Canadian Scholars Press.

Mercer, G. and Berlinger, N. (2020) 'Interdependent citizens: The ethics of care in pandemic recovery', *Hastings Center Report*, 50(3), 56–58.

Mignolo, W.D. (2015) 'Sylvia Wynter: What does it mean to be human', in K. McKittrick (ed), *Sylvia Wynter: On Being Human as Praxis*, Durham, NC: Duke University Press, pp 106–123.

Miller, E.J. and Gwynne, G.V. (1972) *A Life Apart*, London: Tavistock.

Mocarski, R., Eyer, J.C., Hope, D.A., Meyer, H.M., Holt, N.R., Butler, S. and Woodruff, N. (2020) 'Keeping the promise of community-based participatory research: Integrating applied critical rhetorical methods to amplify the community's voice for trial development', *Journal of Community Engagement and Scholarship*, 13(1), 26–35.

Morris, K., Barnes, M. and Mason, P. (2009) *Children, Families and Social Exclusion: Developing New Understandings*, Bristol: Policy Press.

Muñoz, J.E. (1996) 'Ephemera as evidence: Introductory notes to queer acts', *Women and Performance, a Journal of Feminist Theory*, 8(2), 5–16.

Neal, S., Mohan, G., Cochrane, G. and Bennett, K. (2015) '"You can't move in Hackney without bumping into an anthropologist": Why certain places attract research attention', *Qualitative Research*, 16(5), 491–507.

Nussbaum, M. (2001) *Upheavals of Thought: The Intelligence of the Emotions*, Cambridge: Cambridge University Press.

O'Rourke, B. (2018) 'Intercultural encounters as hospitality: An interview with Richard Kearney', *Journal of Virtual Exchange*, 1, 25–39.

Ostrer, C. and Morris, B. (2009) 'First-hand experiences of different approaches to collaborative research' in A. Sweeney, P. Beresford, A. Faulkner, M. Nettle and D. Rose (eds) *This is Survivor Research*, Ross on Wye: PCCS Books, pp 71–81.

Pahl, K. and Facer, K. (2017) 'Understanding collaborative research practices: A lexicon' in K. Facer and K. Pahl (eds) *Valuing Interdisciplinary Collaborative Research: Beyond Impact*, Bristol: Policy Press, 215–231.

Puig de la Bellacasa, M. (2017) *Matters of Care: Speculative Ethics in More Than Human Worlds*, Minneapolis: Minnesota University Press.

Reason, P. (ed) (1994) *Participation in Human Inquiry*, London: SAGE.

Reissman, C.K. (2008) *Narrative Methods for the Human Sciences*, London: SAGE.

Ribbens McCarthy, J., Evans, R., Bowlby, S. and Wouango, J. (2018) 'Making sense of family deaths in urban Senegal: Diversities, contexts and comparisons', *Omega: Journal of Death and Dying*, 82(2), 230–260.

Robinson, F. (2015) 'Care ethics, feminism and the future of feminism' in D. Engster and M. Hamington (eds) *Care Ethics and Political Theory*, Oxford Scholarship Online, doi: 10.1093/acprof:oso/9780198716341.001.0001.

Rodriguez, A.J. and Morrison, D. (2019) 'Expanding and enacting transformative meanings of equity, diversity and social justice in science education', *Cultural Studies of Science Education*, 14(2), 265–281.

Romano, N., Mitchell, V. and Bozalek, V. (2019) 'Why walking the common is more than a walk in the park', *Journal of Public Pedagogies*, 4.

Rose, D. and Beresford, P. (2009) 'Introduction' in A. Sweeney, P. Beresford, A. Faulkner, M. Nettle and D. Rose (eds) *This is Survivor Research*, Ross on Wye: PCS Books, pp 3–10.

Rosiek, J.L., Snyder, J. and Pratt, S.L. (2019) 'The new materialisms and indigenous theories of non-human agency: Making the case for respectful anti-colonial engagement', *Qualitative Inquiry*, 26(3–4), 331–346.

Sander, A. (2021) 'Producing knowledge with care: Building mutually caring researcher-research participants relationship', *Femina Politica*, 70–81, https://doi.org/10.3224/feminapolitica.v30i1.07

Sayer, A. (2011) *Why Things Matter to People: Social Science, Values and Ethical Life*, Cambridge: Cambridge University Press.

Seale, C.F. (1999) *The Quality of Qualitative Research*, London: SAGE.

Sevenhuijsen, S. (1998) *Citizenship and the Ethics of Care: Feminist Considerations on Justice, Morality and Politics*, London: Routledge.

Sevenhuijsen, S. (2003) 'Trace: A method for normative policy analysis from an ethic of care', paper prepared for the Care and Public Policy seminar, University of Bergen, 11 November.

Shakespeare, T. (2000) *Help*, Birmingham: Venture Press.

Simpson, A., Jones, J., Barlow, S. and Cox, L. (2014) 'Adding SUGAR: Service user and carer collaboration in mental health nursing research', *Journal of Psychosocial Nursing and Mental Health Services*, 52(1), 22–30.

Smith, L.T. (1999/2012) *Decolonising Methodologies: Research and Indigenous Peoples*, New York: Zed Books.

Staddon, P. (2012) 'Service user-led research in the NHS: Wasting our time?' in M. Barnes and P. Cotterell (eds) *Critical Perspectives on User Involvement*, Bristol: Policy Press, pp 201–208.

Sweeney, A., Beresford, P., Faulkner, A., Nettle, M. and Rose, D. (eds) (2009) *This is Survivor Research*, Ross on Wye: PCS Books.

Teuber, G. (2006) 'Rights of non humans? Electronic agents and animals as new actors in politics and law', *Journal of Law and Society*, 33(4), 497–521.

Thompson, S. (2006) 'Anger and the struggle for justice' in S. Clarke, P. Hoggett and S. Thompson (eds) *Emotion, Politics and Society*, Basingstoke: Palgrave, pp 123–144.

Tronto, J.C. (1993) *Moral Boundaries: A Political Argument for an Ethic of Care*, New York: Routledge.

Tronto, J.C. (2013) *Caring Democracy: Markets, Equality and Justice*, New York: New York University Press.

Tronto, J.C. (2020) 'Caring democracy: How should concepts travel?' in P. Urban and L. Ward (eds) *Care Ethics, Democratic Citizenship and the State*, Cham: Palgrave Macmillan, pp 181–198.

Tronto, J.C. and Fisher, B. (1990) 'Toward a feminist theory of caring' in E. Abel and M. Nelson (eds) *Circles of Care*, New York: SUNY Press, pp 36–54.

Tsing, A.L. (2015) *The Mushroom at the End of the World: On the Possibility of Life in Capitalist Ruins*, Princeton: Princeton University Press.

Turner, K. and Gillard, S. (2012) ' "Still out there?": Is the service user vice becoming lost as user involvement moves into the mental health research mainstream?' in M. Barnes and P. Cotterell (eds) *Critical Perspectives on User Involvement*, Bristol: Policy Press, pp 189–200.

Vacchelli, E. (2018) *Embodied Research in Migrations Studies*, Bristol: Policy Press.

Vaka, S., Brannelly, T. and Huntington, A. (2016) 'Getting to the heart of the story: Using talanoa to explore Pacific mental health', *Issues in Mental Health Nursing*, 37(8), 537–544.

Visse, M. and Abma, T. (2018) 'Evaluation for a caring society: Toward new imaginaries' in M. Visse and T. Abma (2018) *Evaluation for a Caring Society*, Charlotte, NC: Information Age Publishing.

Visse, M., Abma, T. and Widdershoven, G. (2015) 'Practising political care ethics: Can responsive evaluation foster democratic care?', *Ethics and Social Welfare*, 9(2), 164–182.

Visvanathan, S. (2005) 'Knowledge, justice and democracy' in M. Leach, I. Scoones and B. Wynnes (eds) *Science and Citizens: Globalization and the Challenge of Engagement*, London: Zed Books, pp 83–96.

Walker, M.U. (2007) *Moral Understandings: A Feminist Study in Ethics*, 2nd edn, Oxford: Oxford University Press.

Ward, L. and Barnes, M. (2015) 'Transforming practice with older people through an ethic of care', *British Journal of Social Work*, 46(4), 906–922.

Whittier, N. (2001) 'Emotional strategies: The collective reconstruction and display of oppositional emotions in the movement against child sexual abuse' in J. Goodwin, J.M. Jasper and F. Polletta (eds) *Passionate Politics: Emotions and Social Movements*, Chicago: University of Chicago Press, pp 233–250.

Williams, F. (2001) 'In and beyond New Labour: Towards a political ethic of care', *Critical Social Policy*, 21(4), 467–493.

Williams, F. (2004) 'What matters is what works: Why every child matters to New Labour. Commentary on the DfES Green Paper Every Child Matters', *Critical Social Policy*, 24(3), 406–427.

Williams, F. (2021) *Social Policy: A Critical and Intersectional Analysis*, Cambridge: Polity Press.

Wilson, S. and Wilson, P. (1998) 'Relational accountability to all our relations', *Canadian Journal of Native Education*, 22(2), 155–158.

Wolin, S.S. (1969) 'Political theory as a vocation', *The American Political Science Review*, 63(4), 1062–1082.

Wykes, T. (2014) 'Great expectations for participatory research: What have we achieved in the last ten years?', *World Psychiatry*, 13(1), 24–27.

Wynter, S. (2003) 'Unsettling the coloniality of being/power/truth/ freedom: Towards the human, after man, its overrepresentation – an argument', *The New Centennial Review*, 3(3), 257–337.

Young, I.M. (2000) *Inclusion and Democracy*, Oxford: Oxford University Press.

Young, I.M. (2011) *Responsibility for Justice*, Oxford: Oxford University Press.

Zembylas, M., Bozalek, V. and Shefer, T. (2014) 'Tronto's notion of privileged irresponsibility and the reconceptualisation of care: Implications for critical pedagogies of emotion in higher education', *Gender and Education*, 26(3), 200–214.

# Index

www.ingramcontent.com/pod-product-compliance
Lightning Source LLC
Chambersburg PA
CBHW062108040426
42336CB00042B/2640